Controlling

CROHN'S

DISEASE

Controlling
CROHN'S
DISEASE

The Natural Way

616.3445

Virginia M. Harper
with Tom Monte

KENSINGTON PUBLISHING CORP.
http://www.kensingtonbooks.com

The "Noodles and Broth" recipe on page 202 and "Koi-Kuku" recipe on page 211 are from *Macrobiotic Cooking* by A. Kushi. Copyright © 1985 by Aveline Kushi and Alex Jack. By permission of Warner Books, Inc.

The "Sesame Waffles" and "Apple Syrup" recipes on page 205 are from *The Self-Healing Cookbook*, Fourth Edition, by Kristina Turner. Copyright © 1989 by Kristina Turner. By permission of Kristina Turner.

TWIN STREAMS BOOKS are published by

Kensington Publishing Corp.
850 Third Avenue
New York, NY 10022

Contents

*To my grandmother, whose loving guidance
still surrounds me.
To my parents, who taught me the spirit of family harmony
and that through love all change is possible.
To my children, who were, and continue to be, my inspiration.
You are the beginning of all that I am, the seed for all that I
may become, and the beacon for my eternity.*

Acknowledgments

I wish to thank all of those people who inspired, motivated, and supported the writing of this book.

My brother, Alex, and sister, Maritza, whose love has sustained me through sickness, health, laughter, and tears.

Chip, for loving me the best you knew how and for being with me during the hardest phase of our lives.

Dana, whose dedication to the long hours of interviewing gave this project flight. Your humor kept me smiling.

Dan, for giving the dream the spark of reality.

Sarto, whose friendship, love, and tenacity brought this book to fruition.

Clark, for your wisdom, which helped me get through my growing pains, and for your undying confidence in me.

Ginger, the redheaded angel whose love and friendship have no bounds. You epitomize "best friend." Your patience in reading and rereading the manuscript is greatly appreciated.

Margaret, my mentor, whose loving encouragement and excitement gave energy to my goal.

Jan, for unselfishly giving up your time to type and for your faith in my work.

Crystal, for donating your beautiful God-given talent and for your friendship.

Katherine, the unexpected surprise. You came into my life at the precise moment I needed your help to fulfill my dream. Thank you for your flexibility and ability to read my handwriting.

Todd, whose generous talents made me look good.

Michio and Aveline Kushi, whose vision of and dedication to achieving a peaceful world redirected my life.

Gregg and Michelle, who fed me physically and spiritually. Your guidance and encouragement to teach has given me confidence in my life path.

Mark, my soul mate, whose sincere love, support, and patience have given me the freedom to connect with my spirit and soar. I am enjoying the dance.

Gayle and Peter, whose constant encouragement and help with research are appreciated and invaluable. Gayle, you are the true essence of a diligent spirit.

Tom Cassone, who helped me through the confusion. Strong friendships and memories are forever.

Betty and Diane, whose generosity with information and continuous support have been greatly appreciated.

Beverly, whose undying support has been my buoy through this project. Marriage made us family, experiences made us bond, and divorce made us true friends.

Tom Monte, last but most important, whose dedication and patience are surpassed only by your talented writing skills. You expressed my passion to create my destined project.

All the many other friends and family that have allowed me to be a part of your lives. You have supported me financially, emotionally, and spiritually.

Because of you, my way is made easy.

Foreword

Twenty-five years ago, I met with the dean of one of the nation's top medical schools to ask him to consider funding for a small research project. As a teacher and counselor of hundreds of people who were facing life-threatening, degenerative illness, I had witnessed a significant number of remissions and reversals of grave conditions as a result of simple dietary and lifestyle changes. With more than $80 million in his research war chest that year, the dean had the power to recommend that a small study be undertaken to determine if these anecdotal successes showed any future promise.

I began the meeting by stating my assumptions: that diet played a crucial role in the development of most degenerative diseases, especially cancer of the breast and colon, and that as major killers, these diseases might also be preventable with changes in diet and lifestyle. Responding to the specifics of my hypothesis after a brief, disdainful jaw clenching, this esteemed researcher and scholar dismissed my conclusions as being overly simplistic.

"If you are suggesting that our daily diet of meat, cheese, butter, eggs, sugar, and diet sodas contributes in any way to the development of these diseases," he said, "then you are wasting my time. These illnesses are very complicated, and they are most likely caused by viruses." At the time, the widely held belief that cancer was a virus was the very cornerstone of research.

"Then, how will your research monies be spent?" I asked.

"More research is needed in nuclear medicine, surgery, radiation, and chemotherapy. These are the only ways we can cure these diseases." Prevention wasn't even a possibility, so treatment occupied most of his thoughts. The impatient physician cut our meeting short, granting me only the slight possibility that nitrates in hot dogs may cause some problems. I left disappointed, although no less determined to stay the course. Although I had no more ability to predict the future than he did, I would never have guessed how quickly things would begin to turn around.

In little more than five years, this same man cochaired a prestigious national panel that concluded that diet plays a key role in the majority of cancers in both men and women, catapulting nutritional research into the lead as the focus of promising research for both treatments *and* prevention. A few years later, after the virus theory was abandoned, dozens of other groups reached a similar conclusion: that our daily diet might very well be at the root of our troubles.

Like Pogo, who said, "We have met the enemy, and the enemy is us," many observers could actually find something to celebrate. We could take control—self-navigate—and with care and common sense, not only prevent degenerative illness, but actually treat many cancers with diet as a *primary therapy*. Despite negative reports of extreme treatments and last-ditch efforts to reverse degenerative disease, many patients began to request more information about alternatives, dietary changes, and methods that might complement conventional approaches. The wisest doctors, recalling their Hippocratic oath to do no harm, became compassionate supporters of patients who had little chance of recovery from devastating illnesses. One famous physician, Robert Mendelsohn, known as the People's Doctor, even stated that patients might consider suing doctors who did not inform them of the alternatives to conventional care. Protocols of cancer treatments did little to relieve suffering. A few doctors spoke out against the tide of unproven options, arguing that until more research was done, it was unethical to put forward "false hopes." But by the mid-1990s, the majority of patients with malignancies had already incorporated some alternatives into their daily regimen, giving birth to the new field of "integrative medicine," now widely practiced worldwide.

Amid this revolution in medicine, some people quietly went about the business of healing themselves. Health food stores blossomed, self-help books became bestsellers, and reports of miraculous recoveries by superstars and ordinary mortals filled the airwaves. As a longtime macrobiotic teacher and counselor, I personally saw thousands of people with every devastating disease imaginable, from asthma to metastatic uterine cancer. In nearly every case, diet was clearly a key factor in cause. But never was that more obvious than in the diseases of the digestive system such as Crohn's disease. Years of ingesting processed and refined foods, acidic vegetables, and simple sugars took their toll on tens of thousands of patients. Unbelievably, conventional approaches did little if anything to reverse this condition as patients were sentenced to a shortened lifetime of steroids and suffering.

The Chinese characters that signify crisis also mean opportunity. This paradox remains buried deep in the gut of a beautiful family from Chile. Following the ravages of a poor diet since immigrating to the United States 20 years earlier, one of their own developed severe diarrhea and abdominal pains. When she was eventually diagnosed with Crohn's and placed on prednisone, both she and her family were unwilling to accept that this special woman could not find a way to reverse the degeneration.

Meeting Virginia and her father, Julio, nearly 20 years ago was one of those invaluable experiences that bring such joy to my work. I feel very blessed to have played even a small role in their care, offering some simple guidance and support. But as you read the remarkable story of recovery that follows, know that the clinical approach and specific treatments employed were secondary to what really made a difference in this case. This family was infused with a unity of spirit that is nothing short of unconditional love. And with this love, Virginia Harper was able to un-lock the real secret behind the macrobiotic approach: that be-yond grains, vegetables, and external treatments; beyond acid, alkaline, and azuki beans; macrobiotics is *a way of life*. It is a way of harmony, balance, and unity with our environment, both inner and outer, a sort of unity of spirit that the universe offers each human being from every culture, from every walk of life, no matter what their age or condition. It is nature's expression of unconditional love—restorative, regenerative, and quite simply miraculous.

This book will change your life not just because of the story it tells or the lessons it teaches. This book will burn a hole through the densest firewall of protection around your heart. It will crack open the possibility of recovery from yet another "incurable" dis-ease full of suffering that can be eliminated. This story emerges from the courageous power and commitment of a single soul so determined to find the truth that nothing stood a chance of defeating her. Whether medical school deans or internists take another two decades to arrive at the simple truth of the relation-ship between disease and our way of life won't make any differ-ence now that you have been moved to take control over your own destiny with this book.

Delight in the reality that everything changes, and may your life be filled with the most fortunate blessings!

William Spear
Litchfield, Connecticut
June 2001

Preface

This book offers people with Crohn's disease, ulcerative colitis, and other forms of inflammatory bowel disease (IBD) a program that can fully restore their overall physical and intestinal health. People who are severely ill, as I was, can make a full recovery. By this I mean that people who follow the program described here—and follow it properly—can eliminate the presence of underlying illness. You can live free of all IBD symptoms, as I do. In addition, you can gain tremendous energy, vitality, and clarity of mind. In short, this program can give you back your life.

This book tells the story of my own recovery from severe and advanced Crohn's disease. It also describes in detail the program that saved my life. I also provide recipes and an array of healing behaviors that can encourage healing. As you will see by reading Part One of this book, my illness was so advanced that I was scheduled to use the most powerful chemotherapy agents available and, shortly thereafter, was expected to undergo surgery to remove a portion of my diseased small intestine. If I had followed that course, I would have eventually lost much of my intestinal tract and been forced to undergo an ileostomy, an operation to divert fecal waste through an opening in the intestinal wall.

Instead of following the medically prescribed course of treatment, I adopted a diet and lifestyle known as macrobiotics. For me, this approach to healing was both foreign and extremely challenging. It took time for me to learn how to prepare foods with which I was unfamiliar. It also took time for my palate to adjust, especially to certain foods that I found strange and unappealing. Eventually, I learned how to prepare these foods so that they were delicious and fully satisfying—far more satisfying, in fact, than the standard American diet that I had followed for most of my life. I follow a macrobiotic lifestyle today for the sheer pleasure of it, though I must admit that if I went back to my old ways of eating and lifestyle habits, my illness very likely would return. If this were not the case, however, I would still follow the macrobiotic lifestyle, which has now become my normal way of eating and living.

As I describe in Part One of this book, the diet I initially followed was very restrictive. It had to be. Anyone with Crohn's disease or colitis knows that your choice of foods—even before starting a healing diet—is limited, at best. The reason for the limitations is that the intestines are so diseased that they cannot tolerate a wide array of foods. The wrong foods can cause tremendous suffering.

Most people who suffer from some form of IBD know in their heart that food is a trigger and very likely a cause of the illness. We know this because when we eat certain foods, we experience a rapid onset of symptoms, which can include diarrhea, fever, cramping, pain, and significant blood loss. Many people also believe that they are genetically susceptible to the illness. Indeed, there very likely is a genetic component to IBD. But like cancer, heart disease, and adult-onset diabetes, no IBD can arise unless we create the environmental conditions that promote the expression of that particular gene or set of genes. The primary environmental influence that gives rise to Crohn's or colitis or other IBDs is diet. The typical American diet—the diet most medical doctors encourage you to follow—is causing the slow destruction of your intestinal tract. It is also the reason for tremendous suffering.

After many years of pain and torment from Crohn's disease, I adopted a macrobiotic diet, as described in this book. I did this against the wishes of my doctor, who at times was adamantly opposed to my choice. My doctor's advice, which was based on the recommendations of the American medical establishment, was to eat a standard American diet and continue to take the medications he prescribed. Eventually, I would need surgery, which would result in the gradual loss of my intestines and, eventually, the loss of my rectum. That consequence would require surgeons to create a hole in my abdomen that would allow waste to be eliminated from my body by flowing into a bag that would be strapped to my side.

This is the fate doctors are encouraging their patients with IBDs to accept. It's true that not all people with IBDs fall victim to that fate; some endure their entire lives on various kinds of medications, most of which have life-altering side effects. Anyone with IBD faces a future that is pretty bleak, especially if you accept the medically prescribed path of treatment.

There is another way: the way described in this book. If my experience has taught me anything, it is that few things, if any, are impossible to the human spirit. The old cliché, "Where there is a will, there is a way," is fundamentally true about life. For those who are suffering from Crohn's disease, colitis, or another IBD, the approach described in this book can be that way.

Introduction

Never place a period where God has placed a comma.

—Gracie Allen

The four physicians sat on the podium, sagelike under the bright glow of ceiling lights that illuminated the large hotel banquet room. Each took a turn at describing a pharmaceutical drug, a family of drugs, or a surgical procedure designed to treat Crohn's disease and ulcerative colitis. Their words held an unmistakable enthusiasm that fell on the 200 men, women, and children in the audience like so many broken promises. We were clearly restive. Nothing that had been said sounded particularly new, much less like an effective treatment. The doctors themselves admitted that there was no cure for Crohn's or colitis, nor was there anything like a cure on the immediate horizon. The best anyone could hope for was that the illness might be "managed." That was the operative word. But after suffering not only from the chronic distress of Crohn's—with its stabbing intestinal pains, cramps, and bloody stools—as well as the debilitating side effects of the treatment, I, for one, failed to see the relevance of the word. I also saw little reason for enthusiasm.

The year was 1995, the place, the Stouffer Renaissance Hotel in downtown Nashville, Tennessee. The ostensible reason for the presentation was to bring people who suffered from Crohn's or colitis up to date about the latest advances in treatment. However, what soon became apparent was that the doctors were there to encourage people in the audience to either take the available medications or have surgery. Like so many in the audience, I had learned firsthand that the drugs could be considered only temporary stop-gap measures. Moreover, their debilitating side effects made them a "damned-if-you-do, damned-if-you-don't" proposition. Surgery, whose purpose was to eliminate lengths of diseased intestine, offered even darker side effects.

Unlike everyone else in the audience, I had not come here for answers to these illnesses. I had already been cured of the "incurable."

A lectern and microphone had been placed at the front of the room, directly before the doctors. One by one, people from the audience went to the mike to describe their intense physical distress and their frustration with both the illnesses and the medications. Though each story was unique in its personal details, the general outline was common to most of us in the room.

The Grim Picture of Crohn's and Other IBDs

Once you are afflicted with either Crohn's or colitis—the two conditions have so much in common that even doctors have trouble distinguishing one from the other at times—it becomes the center of your life. It measures out how much energy you have for your chores and for interacting with your loved ones. It decides the kind of day you have—a good day usually means that your symptoms are mild or absent, while a bad day could mean that you must be hospitalized with uncontrollable pain, diarrhea, and dehydration. Once a Crohn's attack occurs, you are doubled over with intestinal pain. You spend hours on the toilet, often with bloody diarrhea. You can keep nothing in your stomach. In many cases, your only choice is to go to the emergency room, where the doctors often run a series of intrusive tests—upper and lower gastrointestinal (GI) series, perhaps, and sometimes even a colonoscopy—to determine that, yes, this is a Crohn's flare-up and you have to be hospitalized for a week to ten days.

During your hospital stay, you are fed intravenously while the open sores in your intestinal tract heal and the inflammation subsides. Eventually, the hospital staff gives you a soft diet of Jell-O, potato soup, and milk—a regimen that brings to mind the cuisine at a Third World prisoner camp. Finally, you are sent home, wounded and weak. It's not uncommon for people with Crohn's or colitis to make six or more hospital visits per year.

More than 1 million Americans suffer from Crohn's disease or ulcerative colitis, illnesses collectively termed inflammatory bowel disorders, or IBDs. Crohn's disease affects the small intestine, an organ that on average is about 22 feet long and is responsible for absorbing the nutrients from food into the bloodstream. The disorder causes the layers of tissue within the small intestine to become inflamed. Very often, that inflammation becomes ulcerated, causing exposed wounds to emerge from within the intestinal walls. The most common site for Crohn's to manifest is the lower part of the organ, a section known as the ileum. Rather than affecting the entire organ, the disorder occurs in patches, with diseased and healthy tissue interspersed throughout the intestine. Those patches of illness spread like a malignancy, however, infecting more and more healthy tissue.

Ulcerative colitis usually affects the colon, or large intestine, an organ about six feet long that is responsible for eliminating waste. In contrast to Crohn's, colitis usually affects only the colon's innermost lining, known as the mucosa.

Crohn's can and often does spread to the large intestine, as well. For this reason, both illnesses are often referred to simply as Crohn's.

As for treating the illness, the most commonly prescribed drugs include the aminosalicylates, aspirinlike compounds of which Azulfidine is the most common; the corticosteroids, or steroids, of which prednisone is most commonly prescribed; antibiotics; and immunosuppressant agents. In one way or another, all the drugs attempt to reduce the inflammation and control the symptoms. However, because the pharmaceuticals do not control the spread of the disease, doctors are sometimes forced to surgically remove sections of the intestines to eliminate irreparably damaged tissue. This, unfortunately, does not contain the illness, either. Consequently, repeated surgeries may be needed. For many, this means that more and more of the digestive tract is lost. Eventually, an ileostomy may be performed in which the colon is removed and a part of the small intestine resected so that it protrudes through the wall of the abdomen. That tubelike projection, called a stoma, empties the intestinal waste into a bag, which hangs at the person's waist.

The All-Too-Apparent Suffering

Needless to say, it was a pretty grim picture that was presented to those of us in the audience. As I looked around the room, I could clearly see the effects of the drugs on some of the people in the audience—so many swollen faces and fidgety feet, two common side effects of the antiinflammatories. Prednisone and some of the other pharmaceuticals can cause a high degree of arousal. They raise your level of anxiety and nervous tension. They also cause a raw, burning sensation in the intestinal tract, as if something is going on in your small and large intestine.

As the meeting wore on, more people seemed willing to express their frustration with medical treatment. One woman said, "So you're saying, I'm going to have to live with this? You're saying that I'm going to have to have a bag?"

Others came to the lectern to relate their experiences with diet as a possible cause of the disorder. Several people reported that certain foods seemed to trigger their flare-ups or make them worse. Every time the question of diet came up, however, the doctors dismissed it with generalities. It is important to eat a balanced diet to get adequate nutrition, one doctor said, especially because Crohn's often prevents optimal absorption of the nutrients from your food. Soft foods are better than fibrous ones, said another, because they are easier on the intestinal tract. As for any scientific link between diet and the cause of either of these two disorders, there was none. Nor was there any evidence that any individual foods trigger a flare-up. As the doctors made clear, there is no known cause of Crohn's or colitis. If a particular food bothers you, stay away from it, one doctor patronized. Otherwise, you should be flexible with your diet.

These statements were incredible to many in the audience. It was as if the doctors were talking about diseases that were very different from the ones that tormented those who had gathered here. Perhaps in an attempt to be helpful to each other, a couple of people came up to the microphone and listed specific foods that they believed trigger Crohn's and colitis attacks. The doctors appeared unmoved by their statements. They were anecdotal reports, not scientific evidence. Though technically true, the doctors' words seemed dismissive and made some in the audience more contentious.

During the presentations, I noticed a man in his late thirties sitting across the aisle from me. He fidgeted in his chair, obviously uncomfortable with all that he had been hearing. Finally, he got up and made his way to the lectern. He was heavyset, with dark hair and a large stomach. He wore a white shirt and blue work pants. "My daughter is thirteen and she has Crohn's disease," he said. "You say food has nothing to do with this disease, but every time she has an ice cream sundae, she ends up in the hospital. A lot of people have told you that food affects this illness. Are all these people crazy? Are we just imagining this? I'm her father and it hurts me to see her this way." As he said these words, his voice cracked with emotion. "I think you should pay more attention to the effects of food on the people with this disease." With that, he resumed his seat. People in the audience nodded their heads at him and at one another. The man had captured not only their experience, but also some of the emotions that went with it.

The doctors on the podium affected concern, but the man's words did not change their recommendation. A pediatrician on the panel said, "Well, as we said, nutrition is important, but your daughter is young. She should be able to eat what she wants. Don't restrict her too much."

Upon hearing those words, I could no longer contain myself. I got up and went to the lectern. I realized that I had to be brief, otherwise I might be asked to sit down. I steeled my determination.

There Is Hope

"I was diagnosed with Crohn's fifteen years ago," I said. "I took most of the drugs that you have discussed today, especially prednisone, and I didn't do so well on them. In fact, I suffered most of the side effects that you have mentioned. My whole body swelled up. I gained a lot of weight. I had joint pain, headaches, depression, and a lot of other symptoms." As I spoke, I kept my eyes off the doctors because I was afraid that one of them might give me a look that would rob me of my resolve. Instead, I turned vaguely in the direction of the audience, too nervous to look at anyone directly.

"I stand before you today Crohn's-free. I stopped having symptoms thirteen years ago. I did it all through food and by changing my lifestyle. Like many people here, I found that many foods hurt me. They made my Crohn's symptoms worse, but I didn't understand why. But once I discovered how food affects me and I started to control what went into my mouth, I was able to control my symptoms. And now I stand here symptom-free, pain-free, and drug-free."

I turned to the doctors now. "We are begging you to pay attention to the nutrition part of this. You have not talked about food, except to say that if a food bothers you, stay away from it. But food is the key to overcoming this disorder. After all, our food is what's going into our intestines and that's what's hurting us. I didn't need scientific proof to change my way of eating, because as far as I am concerned, my life and my experience are proof enough for me."

With that, I started back to my chair. All the tension that had been building up in that room seemed to explode into applause. I looked over at my husband, my mother, my sister, and my friend Clark, who had come with me, to see if they had started the applause. But it was obvious that it was the audience, hungry for any hope and answers, that had responded with such exuberance.

The doctors looked at each other, as if silently asking which one was going to respond to me. Finally, one of them said, "We are looking into this side of the disease. We need more research. This is another area that needs to be studied more."

Shortly thereafter, the meeting closed. People came up to me in droves. In fact, more people came up to me than to the doctors. I had a two-page pamphlet that gave the details of my recovery and how people could get in touch with me for more information. I had brought only a half-dozen-or-so pamphlets, never dreaming that there would be such a demand for them now. After a few minutes, all my materials were gone.

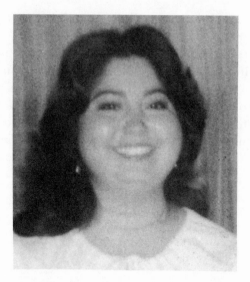

Virginia Harper before meeting William Spear and Michio Kushi (above) and after (below).

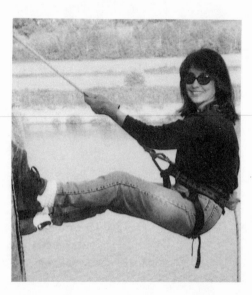

PART ONE

My Story of Recovery

1

Two Life-Altering Diagnoses

I was born in Santiago, Chile, in 1956, and came to the United States in 1963 with my mother, brother, sister, and grandmother. We all joined my father, who had come to the United States the previous year to establish a new life for us in Stamford, Connecticut. My father's first job was as a dishwasher at a restaurant in Greenwich. He had little command of the English language at the time. Looking back, I cannot imagine how difficult it must have been for him as he tried to find work and then hold a job in a foreign land with a foreign culture and a foreign language. It is testimony to my father's courage, intelligence, and sheer strength of will that within a few years of arriving in the United States, he opened his own independent insurance business and turned it into a great success. Like other immigrants, we came to America for the job opportunities and for the possibility of a better life. But my father was the one who paved the way and made it possible for us to realize that dream.

My father, whose name is Julio Marin, was and still is a strong, handsome man. He came from southern Chile, where the people often have light skin and sometimes even blond hair. My father's hair was brown and he wore a mustache, and in his youth he reminded me of the actor Stacy Keach. My father worked long hours and traveled a lot on business. I spent much of my childhood missing him and yearning for his attention. My mother's name is Norma Marin. She came from northern Chile, where the people are darker and their skin more colorful. She was short and stout and always dieting. She was also a great cook, and it was difficult for her to stay away from her own delicious food.

For my mother, America was more a land of mystery and sacrifice than it was of opportunity. After she arrived here, she took a job cleaning hotel rooms. Eventually, she worked as a solderer in an electrical factory, where she remained for many years before retiring. My mother came to see the opportunities offered by America as gifts she gave her children rather than realized herself. Big-hearted, passionate, and full of love, my mother devoted herself to her family. Even though she adopted many American customs, and worked harder than she had ever dreamed she would, her basic values were straight out of the little town where she grew up.

There was always a shadow hanging over her, however, something that she knew and yet fought to keep from thinking about. I didn't realize it until I was a teenager but my father's absences, and more specifically his relationships with other women, had broken my mother's heart. When we were children, she never said a word about his behavior or how much it hurt her. Only after I became a teenager did I realize what was going on, and how she was affected by this secret pain. It would be even later before I realized how much I was affected by it, too.

Despite the difficulties we experienced, our family was filled with love. And of all things I loved as a child, family was the dearest and most important to me. We were a family of only six, counting my grandmother, but ours felt like a big family to me. This was my foundation, my source of love and security. And it was my greatest ambition to be a mother and to have lots of little children running around my house.

I took after my mother in many ways. Like her, I had the more typical Spanish features, including darker skin and hair. I was also short; even my adult height reached only five-feet-two. On the other hand, I inherited my father's trim, athletic body. I grew up playing many different sports, and in junior high and high school,

I swam, played volleyball, ran track, and performed gymnastics, specializing in the uneven parallel bars and floor exercises.

The Mysterious Contradictions of the Physical Body

My body presented me with my most challenging paradox, however. On the one hand, I grew up experiencing tremendous energy, coordination, flexibility, and endurance. On the other, my life has been one long series of health crises. Even when I was a little child, I suffered discomfort in my abdomen. I was chronically constipated, a problem that existed throughout my youth. At age eleven, I developed pain in my right knee that doctors could not diagnose. Later I developed a cyst on my knee and had it surgically removed. At thirteen, I experienced menarche and the foundation of my health suddenly cracked. My menstrual periods were accompanied by torturous cramps, joint pain, and headaches. Midol and other medications made me throw up. My parents could think of nothing to do for me but put me to bed and give me an occasional shot of whiskey. At fifteen, my doctors put me on birth control pills in an attempt to regulate my hormones and diminish my premenstrual syndrome (PMS). The pain only worsened, extending to several days before and after my periods. Soon, it was hard to say if this was PMS anymore. It was simply chronic abdominal pain.

At around fourteen or fifteen, the pain in my abdomen became more intense and localized on the right side of my body. Several more visits to the doctor and a battery of tests revealed nothing, however. My doctors speculated that perhaps I had injured myself on the uneven parallel bars, but they could do little for me.

One day, when I was fifteen, I fainted from the pain in my stomach and lower organs. I was rushed to the hospital, where exploratory surgery was performed. The surgeon removed my appendix, only to find out later that there was nothing wrong with it.

I attended Westhill High School in Stamford and in my sophomore year met a boy named Chip, who would later became my husband. Chip—the nickname was given to him by his parents—was a football player and very popular. With his blond hair and all-American good looks, he resembled a young Robert Redford. He swept me off my feet, and his pursuit of me was intoxicating. Once we became a couple, he was jealous of any boy who would approach me. Perhaps because I grew up with a very controlling father, Chip's behavior did not strike me as controlling or out of the ordinary. On the contrary, I felt loved, desired, and protected.

Steeped in the Spanish culture of Chile, my father enforced his old world view on me and did not allow me to date in high school without the presence of a chaperone. His rules were strict and never questioned. That pitted Chip against my father and there was tension between the two of them from the start of our relationship. Of course, that put me in the middle, which meant that the tension between the two of them was transferred to me. The stress only exacerbated my digestive problems and gave me a constant gnawing sensation in the pit of my stomach.

Finally, in 1974, I graduated from high school. Both Chip and I were accepted at the University of Tennessee (UT), in Knoxville, where he studied business and I studied special education. In fact, Chip and his family were originally from Tennessee. His father was an IBM executive and had been relocated by the big computer business only temporarily to the north. With our acceptance to UT, Chip was essentially taking me to his home.

Despite my physical problems, I tried to live normally and even participated in athletics at UT. I was on the junior varsity swim and gymnastic teams during my freshman year, and also did a life guard certification program. All that swimming, however, caused my right arm to become painful and stiff. Inexplicably, that same arm went numb several times during the summer of 1975. Though the numbness passed, my arm and hand became progressively weaker, to the point that I had trouble holding objects and even lifting my arm. From that point onward, things progressively worsened.

The fall of my sophomore year Chip and I became engaged. A few months later, I found a lump on the right side of my neck. After determining that the lump was a benign cyst, the doctors at the University of Tennessee clinic wanted to remove the mass. However, my parents insisted that I fly home and be seen by my family doctor.

Our family physician, Dr. Octavio Bessa, believed that there was more to this cyst than my Tennessee doctors were saying. Right from the start, he suspected that I had a rare blood disorder called Takayasu arteritis, or "giant cell" arteritis, as it is sometimes called. The illness causes arteries to become inflamed and deformed to the point that the passageway within the artery can narrow and in some cases close entirely. If that closure happens in the neck, it can cause a fatal stroke. If it occurs in an artery that brings blood to the heart, it can cause a fatal heart attack.

Dr. Bessa sent me to several specialists, each of whom rejected his suspicion that my symptoms were being caused by a singular illness, namely Takayasu arteritis. In fact, several dismissed my symptoms as merely emotional. One even patted me on the head and said, "How could a pretty little thing like you be that sick?" Meanwhile, my symptoms worsened. The vision in my right eye became distorted and soon I experienced some blurriness and streaks of silver light that I could only describe as "silver worms." At the same time, my pulse and blood pressure were getting weaker. I was also anemic. It was possible that I was leaking blood from one or more of my arteries.

All the signs pointed to some kind of circulatory disorder, but the doctors could not pinpoint what it was. Finally, at Dr. Bessa's insistence, I was admitted to Stamford Hospital, where I could have an angiogram, a test in which dye is injected into a suspect artery while an x-ray machine monitors the movements of the dye to determine the degree to which the artery is open or closed. A specialist from New York City came up to do the test.

As it turned out, the doctor decided to do two angiograms. The first one was to be on my right carotid artery, located in my neck. The second would assess the condition of my aorta. Both tests were done on successive days in December 1975.

At the Doorstep of Death

The first angiogram was uneventful, although it did show that there was significant obstruction in my right carotid artery. For the second, I would be mildly sedated, even a little high. The second was to assess the condition of my aorta. I had to be sufficiently conscious during the procedure to respond to the doctor's questions. He told me that as the dye moved up into my chest, I would feel a warm sensation. If the dye got hot, he said, I must tell him immediately.

I lay on a table in a laboratory room. A television monitor hung above me to my right. The doctor told me that the monitor would allow us to view what was taking place within me. To inject the dye into my body, a catheter was inserted into my right groin and then moved up through the center of my body and into the aorta. We watched the monitor, which revealed an x-ray image of a catheter wending its way through my thorax. At that point, the dye was released. "Let me know where you feel it," the doctor instructed me in a soothing voice.

I felt the warm dye flow into my chest. It seemed to flood my chest and move upward, toward my neck, around the area of my thyroid. The doctor asked me how the dye felt and I said "warm."

"Let me know if it gets hot," he said again. Meanwhile, he held a stethoscope to my chest and to my neck, around the right carotid artery. The doctor turned to the nurse and said that there was "bruiting" in my neck area and the right side of my chest. The word means abnormal sounds and, in my case, meant that my blood was not flowing properly in these areas.

Suddenly, I felt an intense heat in my neck. "It's hot in my neck," I said. My saliva was red hot. Involuntarily, I let out a loud and deep scream. My voice came from the very center of my being. I kept screaming from this deep place with all the power I had inside me. And then a very odd thing happened. Somehow, I separated myself from my body and literally watched myself in crisis. The terror was so great that I dissociated from my body and became a witness to the events. My body was acting purely on instinct now, in the grip of pure panic. And as I watched myself, I thought, Why am I screaming?

From this detached place, I saw myself go into convulsions. The doctor was frantically calling out codes—he and the nurse were very upset, I realized—as he and the nurse worked to save my life. Something has gone terribly wrong, I thought. Several people rushed into the room. Orders were given to inject me with adrenaline. At the same time, doctors and nurses worked furiously to hold me down.

I was suddenly aware that my tongue was swollen and choking me. I couldn't breathe, but my swollen tongue prevented me from telling anyone. My left arm was being held down by a nurse while a doctor worked feverishly to insert the needle of an intravenous (IV) line. With my free right hand, I grabbed the doctor's wrist and pushed his hand into my mouth in an effort to tell him that my tongue was choking me.

He got the message and yelled out, "She's choking! Give me a clamp!" Suddenly a clamp was inserted into my mouth, depressing my tongue. With that, I passed out.

The next thing I knew, I was on a gurney in the elevator and I was throwing up. A nurse was at my side, helping me turn my head so that I could vomit into some kind of receptacle on the side of the gurney.

"It's okay," the nurse was saying. "It's okay. It happens all the time."

I passed out again but woke up as a couple of nurses attempted to move me from the gurney to the bed in the intensive care ward. I tried to help them by throwing my arms around one of the nurse's neck and holding myself up. But as I did, I realized that my right side seemed heavy and lifeless. I was vaguely aware that I couldn't move my right arm and leg. One of the nurses lifted me, as I clung to her neck with my left hand. My right side hung like so much dead weight. The nurses seemed to realize this, too, because they had to work harder from my right side to get me onto the bed.

Once in the bed, I went to sleep, but when I woke up, I had an intense need to know what had happened to me. I lay there alone for hours, it seemed. I must have been heavily sedated because everything seemed vague and incomprehensible. Finally, they moved me to a regular room.

A nurse came into my room and said that the doctor would be in to see me in a few minutes. I tried to talk to the nurse, but I was incapable of speaking. I was aware that my tongue was extremely thick, but when I tried to speak, I could not form any words. I felt a sudden surge of anxiety that bordered on panic. I wanted my parents to be with me. I also wanted Chip, who was driving from Knoxville to Connecticut to be with me. He had no idea what was happening. Suddenly I had been struck dumb and I desperately wanted someone to tell me what had happened. I also wanted my loved ones to comfort me and tell me that everything would be all right. I struggled to tell the nurse to get my parents, but the only thing that came out of my mouth was some grunting noises.

"Don't strain yourself, honey," the nurse said. "You're going to feel strange for a while."

The nurse left the room and a few minutes later the doctor hurried in. He leaned toward my face and searched my eyes.

"You gave us a scare there, but you're doing well," he said. As the doctor said these words, he behaved in a very upbeat manner that struck me as odd. The thought passed through my mind that perhaps I had done something wrong.

"Do you know your name?" the doctor asked me.

I nodded, but could say nothing.

"Where do you go to school?"

I tried to speak, but no words came out.

"Do you know where you are?"

Again, I nodded affirmatively.

Much to my confusion, the doctor was excited by my answers. "Okay," he said, as if we had just scored a victory. "Where are you?"

Unable to speak, I reached over to the pocket in his lab jacket with my left hand and removed his pen. I motioned that I wanted to write.

"Oh, you want to write," he said. "Okay." He got a pad from the desk and handed it to me.

"I'm okay," I wrote. "What happened to me?"

The doctor looked at the note and was able to read my scribbled writing. His face lit up as if he had just won the lottery. "Oh, this is great," he said. "This is great." Without even so much as a glance at me, he ran out of the room. I would learn later that he ran out to tell my parents that I had not suffered any permanent brain damage. Unbeknownst to me, my parents were waiting outside in the hallway. They were both anxious to see me.

As it turned out, my mother refused to wait for permission to see me. She noticed that the doctors and nurses were pushing a red button that opened the automatic doors to the intensive care ward. When the doctor was preoccupied, she walked up to the doors, pushed the button, and let herself in. Guided only by her intuition, she found my room, walked right up to my bed, and embraced me. Relief overwhelmed me like healing waters.

The next thing I knew, the doctor and my father had joined us. Now the doctor was talking.

"You suffered a stroke," he said. "We didn't know how much brain damage would occur as a result of that stroke. Your loss of speech and the paralysis on the right side of your body are temporary. You'll need some physical therapy but you'll fully recover. You should rest." With that, he was gone and I was finally alone with my parents. They embraced me and we all cried. A few days later, I was released from the hospital and went home.

Finally, a Diagnosis

Once I got home, Chip decided to sit out the next semester to help me through the healing process. I was home about a week when I began speech and physical therapy. Within a month, I was able to talk again, though my annunciation would never be the same. It took a few months, but the paralysis on my right side also passed. I seemed to recover fully, at least in this regard.

Four months after my stroke, in April 1976, doctors at Massachusetts General Hospital in Boston performed an artery graft operation to replace the diseased section of my right carotid artery. The plan was to replace the section of artery with a piece of Dacron material, which would eventually become part of the artery wall. The good news was that if all went well, the material would not restrict my movements or hamper me in any way. The bad news was that the graft had up to only a ten-year life span and would have to be replaced. It would have to be monitored and periodically checked to see if it needed to be replaced. I had just beaten death. Ten years seemed like a long time away.

The surgery lasted four hours. When it was concluded and I opened my eyes, the first face I saw was my surgeon's, who assured me that all had gone well and that I had a very anxious family waiting to see me. Once I was back in my room, my family members all rushed to my bedside. Their love for me poured out of their eyes and smiles. My brother, Alex, broke the intensity of the moment by saying that the doctors had sown my head back on crooked. It hurt my neck to laugh, but no pain had ever felt better.

Later, after they were gone, I looked in the mirror and was immediately horrified. The scar went across my neck. Instead of using stitches, they had used staples in order to keep the scarring down. My right side was swollen all the way up into my face, and the staples made me look like Frankenstein. As tears rolled down my face, I forced myself to be grateful that I was still alive. I glanced out the window at the Charles River, which flowed peacefully, with only a few white caps from the breeze. It was a beautiful, sunny spring day, and children were running alongside the river trying to get their kites airborn. For a moment, I wanted to be one of those kites, free and without any concerns. A heavy feeling gnawed at me that living with Takayasu was only the beginning of the difficulties that lay ahead. As I turned back to examine my face in the mirror, more tears began to roll down my cheeks. "I should be grateful that I'm alive," I told myself. But I wondered if I would ever look the same.

After my family was gone and I had spent some time alone, a Mass General physician told me that I did indeed have Takayasu arteritis. The illness, which has no known cause, is an autoimmune disease in which blood seeps through the artery walls—hence the leakage and related symptoms I experienced. The immune system, which recognizes this leakage as a threat to health, responds by creating inflammation within the artery wall. At the same time, cells within the artery begin to reproduce and create additional tissue, thus further damaging the artery. Eventually, the inflammation and deformed tissue can block the blood flow to the heart, brain, or other organs, possibly causing a fatal heart attack or stroke. My doctors believed that it was exactly this inflammation that was responsible for the diminished blood flow in my right arm, hand, and eye, resulting in my numbness and distorted vision.

There is no cure for the Takayasu arteritis, my doctors told me. The treatment was to put me on a corticosteroid drug, a synthetic steroid called prednisone, to control the inflammation. In addition to the prednisone, I was to take an aspirin every day to thin my blood and thus improve my circulation.

Some part of me was happy that the doctors had finally discovered the cause of my symptoms and grateful for the powers of modern medicine to save me. But it wasn't long before I realized that this was no time to celebrate. In addition to the disease being potentially lethal, the prednisone was cause for concern. My doctors told me that they would have to adjust the dosage of the drug to regulate its side effects. That sounded ominous, but I tried to stay positive. You will have to eliminate all athletic activities, the doctors told me, because the illness prevents optimal blood flow to the heart and other organs. The drug complicates matters, as well, because it is an immunosuppressant, which means that it would slow the healing process after any injury I might suffer. In fact, I would have to eliminate virtually all strenuous activities. Meanwhile, I must pay careful attention to how the drugs affect my body, the doctor told me. I was shocked by all of this. I would have to change my lifestyle entirely. I didn't realize it but he was saving the worst for last.

"You must avoid getting pregnant. It is too risky for you to have children," the doctor told me flatly. The illness could prevent maximal blood flow to the fetus. The drug might cause complications for the developing baby, as well. In all probability, the baby would not survive gestation, and if it did, it might be handicapped as a consequence of my poor health.

It was as if someone had hit me with a baseball bat and I was suddenly seeing stars. I didn't know what to say. I had just been stripped of my womanhood and my most important dream.

"What do you mean, I can't have children?" I said. "Won't the drug keep this illness under control enough for me to get pregnant and give birth?"

"We don't think so. There's no cure for this disease. The best we can hope for is that it can be controlled so that you can live a long, normal life."

Live for what? I thought to myself. Normal in what way? Darkness seemed to fall over me and swallow me whole. What would Chip say? I wondered. He's going to be devastated. He wants a family as much as I do. "There's got to be something you can do," I said to the doctor, no small desperation in my voice.

He just looked at me. "I'm sorry," he said.

Chip took the news hard, but he was unwavering in his support for me and his commitment to our approaching marriage. We had set our wedding date for June 1976, just two months after my diagnosis with Takayasu disease, and neither one of us wanted to change it. We talked for hours about my health problems, what they would mean for our marriage, and about adopting. Yes, we'll adopt, he said. And we'll have the family we both want. He suddenly accepted my problems as his own and accepted the idea that we would adopt children. That was Chip at his best. As the years ahead would prove, Chip had an unbelievable capacity to stay with me through thick and thin. We were about to learn just how thin things were going to get.

A Treatment That Causes More Pain

I was never fully prepared for the side effects of the prednisone. Immediately, my body became swollen, especially around my joints. I developed a moon face and chipmunk cheeks, common side effects among people who take the drug. I was constantly bloated. The drug made me irritable, nervous, and restless. I could not sit still. Two minutes in any one position was more than I could bear. Everything inside of me seemed to be moving to its own rhythm. I felt completely out of harmony inside myself. My skin became overly sensitive and at times I hated being touched. I also developed an insatiable hunger. I could eat a five-course meal and be hungry an hour later. And then I started to gain weight. I had never been overweight in my life; I had always had the self-image of a fit and athletic woman. But now I was a typical overweight housewife, I told myself. I fell into depression, anger, and despair. Look at me, I told myself. Where is my life going? This is just going to get worse. What good could I do, even for my husband? I thought. What value did I have for anyone? Such lines of thinking led to hopelessness and tears.

Somehow, my spirit would overcome the darkness within me. The spark of hope would ignite and burn for a while, but it never lasted long. My emotions became a daily roller coaster ride, but on the whole, I spent a lot more time in the dark valleys than on the light-filled mountaintops.

When I brought up my symptoms to my doctor, he told me that he would adjust the dosage and my body would eventually adapt.

Chip and I were married as planned on June 19, 1976. The effects of the prednisone were already evident in my swollen and puffy cheeks and the dark circles under my eyes. I was far from the image of the beautiful bride. Still, the day was radiant in every other way for me, and for Chip. As far as both of us were concerned, we had the perfect wedding day.

We went on a cruise for our honeymoon. On board the ship, food was everywhere. It was like one of those ancient Roman feasts designed to induce gluttony. The prednisone alone had created an insatiable appetite, but the availability of all that food provided a stimulus all its own. I ate constantly, and by the time we left the ship, I was so overweight that I had to wear my husband's clothes off the boat. None of mine would fit anymore.

Chip and I settled in Tennessee, just outside Nashville. These were Chip's roots and he was overjoyed to start out in his beloved state. I had taken to the South, as well. I loved its slower pace of life, neighborly hospitality, and beautiful country settings. Living in a small town was a new experience for me. Soon we joined a church, built a house of our own, and got to know our neighbors.

It wasn't long before we adopted many of the customs of the South, starting with the Southern diet. Like many of my neighbors, I used lard or butter to cook everything—eggs, bacon, chicken, and meats. Everything had to have lots of grease on it. I made fried chicken, fried steak, fried potatoes, and fried eggs. And if it wasn't cooked with grease, then it had to be sugar-coated. One of the side effects of the prednisone was that I found myself craving sugar, so many of the Southern desserts and snacks became a necessity in my home. One of the desserts that I became adept at making was chess pie, which is made from sugar, eggs, and milk. Between the two of us, Chip and I drank a gallon of milk every week. We loved the Southern diet. Chip would comment regularly that he had never eaten so well in his life as he did when we moved to the South. Of course, this diet just added more pounds to me. Between the bloating, swelling, and weight gain, I was so puffy that I felt that if someone stuck a pin in me, I would burst.

Meanwhile, we also started talking like Southerners. Unconsciously, I developed a slight drawl and picked up the Southern speech patterns. I found myself saying "y'all" and other Southern expressions. Many of my consonants became rounder and softer. But there was a dark side to the changes in my speech patterns, as well.

During the summer of 1976, I realized that the clarity of my speech had not been fully restored, as the doctor who performed the angiograms on me had said it would. On the contrary, I occasionally slurred my words, especially when I was tired, and sometimes I had to struggle to find the right word. The doctor had assured me that all the effects of the stroke would wear off, but that wasn't happening.

Meanwhile, the side effects of the prednisone were getting worse. I developed headaches and terrible night sweats—literally soaked my pajamas and the sheets—and I became increasingly irritable. I suffered from regular bouts of insomnia and my energy levels fluctuated wildly. Sometimes I would have so much energy that I felt as if I could clean several houses, and other times I would be exhausted and depressed and anxious. Depression, anxiety, and elation were tossing me about on a daily basis.

The effects of all these symptoms on my marriage were devastating. "Why did you marry me?" I screamed at Chip. "You don't deserve this. I'm a mess."

Chip never actually dealt with emotions. He came from a family that presented a perfect, upper-middle-class persona. He was of good Southern stock, as he used to say, and in that strata of society, you don't lose control of your emotions and you most certainly do not act out. The drugs I was taking caused periodic emotional outbursts, some of which bordered on hysteria. Rather than deal directly with my issues, however, Chip at first would admonish me to behave—wives don't act in such an immature and un-Christian-like manner, he used to tell me. I was apparently not maintaining the standards of behavior that were expected of a wife in the Bible Belt. Eventually, his tirades would subside, as would my own. At that point, he would become withdrawn and stoical. That only lowered my self-esteem, however, and made me feel insecure about our relationship. I was never sure where I stood with him.

As my weight increased and my emotions became more unstable, I felt increasingly isolated. I went to my doctor for help. His response was to prescribe more drugs, some of which were intended to regulate the effects of the prednisone. I took Azulfidine and potassium, in addition to the aspirin. At the same time, he regulated the dosages of the prednisone. The dosages I took of the prednisone ranged from 10 to 60 milligrams. Eventually, they would get up to 90 mg a day and then to 120 mg daily. It seemed that I was all over the map when it came to the levels of prednisone I took, as well as its varying side effects.

The Lurking Monster Finally Appears

During the early part of 1977, a new set of symptoms arose, or rather an old set returned—and this time with a vengeance. I began to experience severe stomach and intestinal pain. At times, the pain was so sharp that it radiated from the front of my body to the back. It came on without any warning. Suddenly, a stabbing pain would sear through my abdomen, ripple along my back, and double me over. The pain was completely paralyzing. I had to lie down, even if it meant staying on the floor for a few minutes until it subsided enough to allow me to get to my bed. The pain would last anywhere from a few minutes to an hour.

These attacks persisted and grew throughout 1977. Now the pain was radiating throughout my lower and upper body. No pattern seemed to emerge that might suggest a cause. The pain came on days that I ate a great deal as well as on days that I ate very little. It didn't matter what kind of food I ate, or when. Perhaps emotions and stress might have something to do with it, I told Chip. But even my emotions and stress levels could not account for when the pain arose.

I naturally assumed that the attacks stemmed from the Takayasu arteritis. Perhaps blood vessels within my intestines had become inflamed and deformed by the disease, thus triggering the pain. That was the only thing I could think of that might be the cause.

One other related symptom emerged, however, and seemed related to these painful attacks. My digestion, which had always been problematical, was suddenly worse. The chronic constipation was now regularly interrupted by bouts of diarrhea. My doctors performed a wide variety of diagnostic tests, including upper and lower GI series, but nothing proved conclusive.

Finally, in November 1977, all of these symptoms came to a crisis. One day, the pain suddenly stabbed through my intestines and back. I also felt an immediate urge to move my bowels. Much to my horror, the toilet was filled with blood.

I went to the emergency room at Vanderbilt Hospital in Nashville. My first priority upon getting to the hospital was to find a doctor who knew something about Takayasu arteritis. I told the attending physician that I had been diagnosed with this disease and that only a doctor who knew something about it could treat me properly. Soon, a Dr. Jonathan Smith came into the emergency room, introduced himself, and proceeded to diagnose me.

He expressed concern about the bleeding and about the possibility that the Takayasu had affected my aorta, which could be fatal. He did a series of tests, including an upper and lower GI. He could find nothing definitive, however, and soon I was released. However, I liked Dr. Smith and felt comfortable with him.

Between November 1977 and March 1978, I made several trips to the Vanderbilt Hospital emergency room as a result of my abdominal pain and bloody diarrhea. Each time, the doctors fed me intravenously until the inflammation in my intestines subsided. At that point, I got the soft diet of Jell-O and milk. After about a week in the hospital, I would be released to go home, anemic and weak. I lost so much blood during these painful diarrhea attacks that it would take me another week after returning from the hospital to regain my strength.

In March 1978, Chip and I decided to visit his parents, who were living in Great Falls, Virginia, for a vacation. While visiting Chip's parents, we met some old friends. The four of us decided to go to an Italian restaurant for dinner that night. Once in the restaurant, I ordered manicotti shells stuffed with cheese and garlic and covered with spicy marinara sauce. There was wine, salad, and bread, as well. We finished the meal with a dessert of canolis.

That night, we returned to Chip's parents' house and I knew that something was very wrong in my stomach and intestines. It felt as if my intestines were filled with acid. It was a time of closeness, so I ignored the uncomfortable pressure. I did not want to spoil Chip's evening, so I made little of my problems, except to say that the meal didn't sit right with me.

After a few hours, however, I had to get up to go to the bathroom. Again, I filled the toilet with blood. Chip was aghast. He wanted to call his parents, who no doubt were sound asleep, and then take me to the hospital.

"Let's not bother your parents," I said, the fear building inside of me. "Let's just go directly to the hospital."

We went to the emergency room in Fairfax, Virginia. It was a new and very modern hospital. Immediately, the doctors put tubes down my throat and conducted yet another series of tests. I tried to tell them what the problem was and how to treat me, but they ran every test they could think of, or at least it felt that way. In addition to everything I had been given in the past, they also did a barium enema to test my intestinal tract. To do the test, I had to drink a thick solution of barium. The barium absorbs the x-rays and shows the outline of the intestinal tract, thus revealing the condition of the intestines and any abnormalities that might exist. Horrible though it was, the test proved critical because it finally showed what was causing all my intestinal pain and distress.

After all the tests had been done, two doctors entered my room and said that they had discovered my problem. "You have a digestive disorder called Crohn's disease," one of them said. He then went on to explain that Crohn's is caused by inflammation in the small intestine. The bloody stools were caused by open sores in my intestinal tract that were leaking blood. My response surprised them. "You've discovered what I have. That's great," I said. Finally, we knew what the cause of my problems was.

"The good news is that we know how to treat it," the doctor continued. "We use a drug called prednisone, which will control your inflammation."

I was immediately confused.

"But I'm already taking prednisone," I said.

"We know. We're just going to increase your dosage a little to help control this disease."

"But if I'm already taking prednisone, how could I have gotten Crohn's disease in the first place?" I asked them.

The two doctors looked at each other and then at me.

"We don't know the answer to that," one said. There was a pause and then the same doctor began to speak again. "There is no cure for Crohn's disease," the doctor said. "We're not sure what causes the illness. The prednisone will control the symptoms. You and your doctor will have to work together to regulate the dosage over time.

"I must tell you that you should not get pregnant," he continued. "In all probability, your body would not tolerate a pregnancy and you would miscarry. It is best that you avoid getting pregnant at all costs. You can adopt, of course. You and your husband should think about that."

The fact that I had been told before not to have children did not make this latest pronouncement any easier to accept. In fact, it hurt far more than I thought it would. I didn't dwell on those feelings, however, because in that moment there were more immediate concerns pressing on me. What exactly was Crohn's disease? I wondered. Was it related to my Takayasu arteritis? Would the prednisone really control the terrible symptoms I was having? How serious was this illness? Suddenly, the question that I was fighting to keep from my awareness broke through my barricades: Am I dying?

2

The Cruel World of Crohn's Disease

No, I wasn't dying, but such reassurance did little to allay my fears, especially when I learned more about Crohn's disease. As I lay in my hospital bed, my mind struggled to make sense of the obvious contradiction surrounding the prednisone. I kept wondering how I could get Crohn's disease when I was already taking a drug that was supposed to treat the illness and prevent its symptoms. It didn't make sense to me. As soon as Chip and I returned to Tennessee, I began to research these two life-threatening conditions that plagued me. I was a student at George Peabody College at Vanderbilt University. I had access to the medical library there. I buried myself in the medical journals, and with each line I read, I realized my life sentence. The illness was located in my ileum, the final section of the small intestine that ultimately joins with the large intestine. It is within the ileum that most of the nutrients in our food are absorbed into the bloodstream. Unlike ulcerative colitis, which affects only the first or innermost layer of the large intestine, Crohn's disease transforms all the layers of the small intestine into inflamed, diseased tissue and open sores. The result is a variety of symptoms, including loss of appetite, diarrhea, cramps, abdominal pain, fever, and rectal bleeding, symptoms I had already suffered many times in my life. As I had just experienced, they could become so severe that I would have to be hospitalized and fed intravenously until my intestines healed. Crohn's and ulcerative colitis are the two most common inflammatory bowel disorders. More than 1 million Americans suffer from one or both of these illnesses.

There is no cure for Crohn's disease, nor for ulcerative colitis, but there are several drugs that treat the illness, prednisone being the most widely prescribed. Unfortunately, these drugs do not stop the disease from "traveling" to other parts of the small intestine. Many people with Crohn's are left with no alternative but to have lengths of their small intestine surgically removed. The remaining parts are then joined, or "resected." Even the surgery does not stop the disease from spreading, which means that numerous operations may be needed. Eventually, the person may have little remaining of his or her intestines or colon. For many people, the spread of the disease requires an ileostomy, a surgical procedure in which the large intestine is removed and a section of the small intestine is made to protrude through the abdomen wall, where waste is eliminated into a small bag that hangs around the waist. That was the terrible and terrifying future to which I could look forward.

What troubled me even more was that I had been told again not to become pregnant and have children—this for the second time: once for the Takayasu arteritis and now for the Crohn's. The doctors assured me that the Takayasu disease would very likely cause a miscarriage, but if the baby went to term, I might not survive the pregnancy or the birth. The reason: The stress of the pregnancy and the change in my hormonal environment might cause my arteries to become so inflamed and blocked that I could suffer a stroke or a heart attack. There was also the possibility that these same symptoms would deprive the fetus of sufficient blood and oxygen to grow normally, and thus cause some sort of deformity.

Now, on top of the Takayasu disease was the Crohn's. Why did that prevent me from having children? I asked. The answer: the prednisone. It was very likely that I would be on that drug for the rest of my life. No one knew what the effects of the drug would be on me, much less on a baby, but the best guess anyone could give me was that I would probably miscarry. If I didn't, the chances were very high that I would give birth to a severely handicapped child.

Why had I been deprived of the thing I wanted most? I kept asking God. This couldn't be my fate. As I sat there paralyzed by the information, surrounded by the endless walls of books, I thought of my family. More than anything else in the world, I loved my family and dreamed of one day creating my own. We were a big, passionate Spanish family that loved to sing and dance and quarrel and make up. Even though my mother and father had had only three children themselves, we weren't just five people, but six, thanks to the fact that my father had brought his mother to the United States to live with us. His two sisters lived in Stamford as well, not far from our home. We eight were a family, with my grandmother at the center.

Contrary to what might be expected, my mother and grandmother got along beautifully. They loved, respected, and even admired each other, and I always knew why. Both were strong women, drawn from the same ancient Chilean soil, and shared the kind of resolute commitment to family that you rarely see anymore. My grandmother's husband had died when my father was just a boy, which meant that my grandmother had had to keep her family together as a single mother. My mother kept her family together, even in the face of my father's absences and her loneliness. Despite the pain that caused her, she never lost her beautiful smile, nor her loving heart. Anyone who ever met my mother marveled at her capacity to understand, to tolerate, and to hold all her burdens with equilibrium and even a certain joy. I attributed these characteristics to her natural strength and deep spirituality, which she shared with my grandmother.

My grandmother had a strong, Spanish face and a great spiritual presence. Occasionally, I would walk past her bedroom at night and see her on her knees, praying in a whisper beside her bed. Sometimes I would kneel down at her side and pray with her. At that moment, her voice would grow a little louder, so that I could hear her words. She was praying for me, I suddenly would realize. Drawn into her powerful, mysterious world, like a satellite pulled into orbit around a planet, I would experience some hint of her spiritual intensity. Her prayers were so rich and mysterious, they seemed to draw God into her world. When I got up to leave, I always peered back at her with wonder and awe. For her part, my grandmother would remain unfazed by my slipping away; the only small change in her bearing would be the resumption of her whisper, as she plunged ever more deeply into her inner world. Her prayer, it seemed, would go on endlessly.

In many ways, she and my mother were two of a kind, a very rare kind, it seemed to me. By their dignity and love, they made it clear to me that the women in our family were strong and committed, even mysterious, which seemed to give them special powers. These two were my heroes early in life. It seemed natural to me that one day I too would be a mother, like them. There was nothing I wanted more.

But now, for the second time in my life, I was being told by doctors not to even consider motherhood. To ensure that I avoid pregnancy, my doctors eventually inserted an intrauterine device (IUD). I felt like a failure and was bitterly disappointed. Surely my life was meant for more, I said to myself. I felt so powerless. My thoughts were racing. I couldn't breathe. I felt as if the library cubicle was closing in on me. I sobbed over the words that outlined my future. Hours passed, but it didn't seem to matter. Life seemed frozen. I walked outside to my car and resented the life going on around me. The beautiful day seemed to mock me. In light of my illness, I immediately withdrew from school.

Treatment Without Cure

I was newly married, but the part of my life that would soon preoccupy me would not be my husband, but my illness.

My doctors increased my dosage of prednisone. I continued to take the Azulfidine and the potassium. The relatively low dose of prednisone that I had been taking for the Takayasu disease had already caused swelling throughout my body as well as weight gain. Now, with the increased dosage, my weight shot up dramatically and I experienced a host of new symptoms. My face got puffy; my joints swelled; my moods swung from manic highs to painful depressions. I was always nervous and restless inside. Something inside of me couldn't relax, it seemed. I craved carbohydrates, especially sugar, and soon became addicted to pastries, doughnuts, and other sweets. Some mornings when I woke up my ankles would be so swollen that I would have to sit on the edge of my bed and test them to see if they could hold up my weight.

In addition to these symptoms, which seemed more related to the prednisone than the Crohn's disease, were the symptoms of the illness itself. Diarrhea was a daily occurrence. Fatigue, cramps, and stomach pain—these, too, were part of the routine fabric of my life, even the norm. The really intense trouble, however, came when I suffered from one of my flare-ups. My flare-ups varied in intensity. Sometimes a flare-up would last only a few hours; at other times, it would last for days. The worst would land me in the hospital for up to a week. I couldn't be certain how bad a flare-up would be until it had finally run its course. Typically, it started with a severe bout of diarrhea—two or three such attacks within a two-hour period. These attacks might last through the day. Meanwhile, I would be stabbed by intense cramps, gas, and abdominal pain. A fever might emerge. Usually, I would have blood in my stools, and if the flare-up was particularly bad, I would bleed a lot. The blood loss not only would terrify me, but would drain me of my energy and strength. I would feel as if the life force had run out of me. Once a flare-up occurred, I would be bedridden for three or four days.

I drank Maalox by the gallon, it seemed, hoping the diarrhea would let up, but once a flare-up began, there was no stopping it until the storm had passed of its own accord.

At first, I could not find any pattern to the flare-ups—they came and went without rhyme or reason, or so it seemed to me. But later I realized that they were always more frequent and intense in the fall, beginning in September and lasting well past the holidays. During the fall months, I would suffer at least two flare-ups a month, which meant that I would be bedridden for most of the season.

If a flare-up became uncontrollable and the symptoms sufficiently intense, I would be forced to go to the hospital. There I would be fed intravenously until my intestines healed sufficiently to tolerate soft foods, such as potato soup, Jell-O, pudding, and milk.

In the spring of 1978, just after I had been diagnosed, I did my best to cope with the effects of the medication, the daily suffering from the Crohn's, and the regular flare-ups that forced me to bed. I was not the only one dealing with these symptoms, of course. My husband, Chip, was doing his best to support me, but my condition altered both our lives. Though Chip had originally matriculated at the University of Tennessee, he transferred to David Lipscomb College in Nashville. We moved to a duplex on the campus. We were very involved in our Church of Christ community, which held all kinds of social events throughout the year. The thing that determined whether we could attend any particular social event, however, was my health. If I was not experiencing the kind of control over my bowel movements that gave me some semblance of confidence, I could not attend an event. Sometimes Chip would go by himself, but most of the time he would remain home with me.

An Unexpected Miracle

One morning in June 1978, I felt faint and light-headed while I was in the shower. I immediately turned off the water and got out, but the light-headedness became more intense. I realized that I might pass out at any moment so I sat down on the floor. Chip came into the bathroom and saw me, wrapped in a towel and doubled-over on the floor.

"You're white! What's wrong?" he said.

"I don't know," I said. "I feel like I'm going to faint. I think I'm going to throw up."

Suddenly I knew. "Oh my God, I wonder if I'm pregnant." "No," said Chip, "you can't be pregnant. You've got an IUD." But something inside of me knew the truth. "I think I'm pregnant," I said. "You better go get a pregnancy test."

Chip left immediately for the drug store and within 20 minutes was back in our bathroom. As instructed, I peed in a small container and inserted a paper stick. I then placed the test on a little shelf in my bathroom and went out of the room. We would know our fate in fifteen minutes.

Chip and I sat on the couch in our living room and waited for that little slip of paper to divine the future. We sat in silence, holding hands. Whenever Chip and I were together and he didn't know what to do, he held my hand. It was a sweet, vulnerable thing to do. Now, as we sat on the couch together, we were nervous, even afraid. Neither one of us knew what to do, so we held hands and waited.

When the 15 minutes were up, I walked into the bathroom. Chip followed behind me. I went over to the paper stick, picked it up, observed the color, and handed it to Chip. I burst into tears. I was pregnant.

What did I feel first? Which emotions followed that initial feeling? I cannot answer. I felt everything at once. Joy, fear, and misery. If it's possible to shoot skyward with elation and, at the same time, sink into the bottom of one's being with fear, shame, and even anger, I managed it at that moment. All of my conflicting emotions overwhelmed me and spilled out.

What was my fate and my baby's now? I had been warned by my doctors not to get pregnant. The warning was clear: Become pregnant and you risk killing yourself and your baby. At minimum, you may give birth to a severely handicapped child. I had respected that warning. I acquiesced when they advised me to have an IUD inserted. Why hadn't the IUD prevented me from becoming pregnant? How could it fail? But it had failed, and now here I was facing all the dangers my doctors had warned me of.

They had told me that if I became pregnant, I very likely would have to abort the child. I did not believe in abortion and the very thought of it threw me into terrible conflict. For me, abortion was killing a child. There were no "buts" or "what ifs" on that question. But if I didn't have an abortion, I might kill myself and the baby. Was my intense desire to allow the pregnancy to go forward tantamount to suicide? How certain were my doctors that I absolutely needed an abortion? I wondered. Couldn't I risk the pregnancy? What was this pregnancy going to do to my physical, emotional, and spiritual life? I kept wondering.

There was another feeling lurking below the fear, one that was less obvious than the physical fear and the spiritual conflict, but palpable nonetheless. I distinctly felt as if I had done something wrong. My doctors had ordered me not to become pregnant, but I had gone against their order—not by my own volition—but by an accident of nature. Some part of me felt as if I had been a bad girl and I was suffering pangs of guilt and shame. I was angry that I should feel something so stupid and irrelevant, but I could not avoid it. What would my doctor say when I gave him the news? I wondered.

All of that was the dark side of my being. But even in the face of this pain and torment, elation and excitement exploded in me, too. Perhaps it was the woman in me that was celebrating, the woman who longed to become a mother. In some quarter of my being, I was fulfilled, happy, and even justified. I wasn't as physically weak as my doctors had led me to believe. Even with the IUD, I had become pregnant. Wasn't that some kind of miracle?

But I couldn't let myself be happy; I couldn't celebrate in the way that I wanted to. Every time I let myself experience just a hint of happiness, all those other emotions crowded into my consciousness. There was no place inside me where I could rest emotionally, no place where I could feel certain, committed, or free of conflict.

Assaulted by all those competing emotions, all I could do was cry. All of my confusion, fear, and happiness came out in tears.

That afternoon, I called Dr. Smith. Contrary to what I had expected, he was very calming and reassuring.

"Okay," he said. "This was not what we were expecting, but don't worry. I'll get you set up with an obstetrician and we'll work out a plan." He assured me that a lot could be done for me and that he would arrange for me to meet an obstetrician who specialized in high-risk pregnancies. "We're going to do everything we can," he said.

I was surprised and relieved by Dr. Smith's attitude toward me and my pregnancy. He was not overly alarmed, nor was he in any way critical of me.

Next I called my parents to tell them the news. My mother knew very well the dangers surrounding any pregnancy I might have and she reacted as I expected, with care and love.

"Oh, *mi hijita*," she said, which means "my little daughter" in Spanish. That phrase can mean so many different things, depending on the tone of voice. It can be used in celebration or in concern, and there was no doubt now that my mother was feeling the latter.

"I don't know what to say, *mi hijita*," she said. "Look at the situation you're in. We must leave it in God's hands. Don't try to figure it out right now. God will lead you to your answer." My parents insisted that I not forget our native language, so even as I learned English, I spoke Spanish with them. I felt a certain reassurance in being able to speak with them in our language.

My father expressed similar concerns, but he was also reassuring. That was my father. For all his faults, he was a man of great love, great passion, and steadfast in the face of any sort of trouble. Like my mother, my father was completely committed to his children. "You are going to be all right," he told me. "We're going to find the best people and you're going to be fine."

When I got off the telephone with them, I felt terribly sad. That call should have been filled with elation and family celebration, but instead the news had brought worry and fear. Darkness had eclipsed the light.

After I spoke to my parents, Chip called his family. They were not emotional people. They always held their feelings in check. His mother's first words were, "Oh no." Then she paused, as if to find the neutral ground again. "Well," she said, "let's see what the doctor is going to say after he sees her."

After we had spoken to our families, Chip and I went for a

walk in a nearby park. It was a spectacular day in June. The sun poured down a young summer heat, holding us in its secure embrace. Chip was never one to say a lot of deep things to me, and under the circumstances neither of us knew what to say. We walked for a while in silence, holding hands. Finally, we started talking about the possibility of terminating the pregnancy. My doctors had told me that the pregnancy would likely cause the Takayasu arteritis to worsen, which could cause a stroke or a heart attack. I had already had a stroke and was terrified of having another. In addition, the prednisone could cause the child to be deformed. It was possible that the baby would naturally abort if the deformity was too severe, but both of us knew that if we decided to go ahead with the pregnancy, we would do all we could to keep the child alive.

We both agreed that the only way I would have an abortion was if the doctor was certain that the pregnancy would kill me. If the chances were good that I would survive, we would go ahead and give birth to our baby. In that case we would have to face the other likely eventuality, that our child would be handicapped.

Finally, Chip said, "Well, it seems like we're meant to have this baby, because God has prepared you for it."

He was referring to the fact that I had always loved to work with handicapped children and had been studying special education in college. "This pregnancy and these circumstances seem meant to be," Chip said. "God must know you can handle it."

Chip's words turned the tide. From that moment, our attitudes toward the pregnancy and our baby changed from fear to a full embrace. It was as if, by acknowledging the presence of a higher power in this process, Chip had made us part of something larger, benevolent, and supportive. Somehow things would turn out right, we suddenly believed. Neither one of us knew how such a thing might happen, but we had faith. And in any case, he was right: I had been prepared for this moment and this child. The fact that the IUD had failed seemed only to confirm that God had plans of His own for us. From that moment on, we both agreed that if the doctor could give me a good chance of surviving, we would go ahead and have this baby.

That night I lay in bed and tried to pray. I didn't now how. What should I say to God? Was this a gift or was I going to need an abortion? I decided not to allow myself to think of fearful things. I was not going to consider outcomes just yet. Finally I said to God, "Whatever You want this to be, let it be." The words had come to me spontaneously, but no sooner had I said them than I realized that this was something my grandmother would say. That knowledge gave me a certain peace and even a little pride. My grandmother was strong and had deep faith. God had carried her through life, as He would me.

Choosing Life

A few days later, I saw Dr. Smith, who immediately made it clear to me that a termination of the pregnancy would be a medical abortion. I told him that if it was possible, I wanted to go ahead with the pregnancy. He then gave me the name of an obstetrician who specialized in high-risk pregnancies. I immediately made an appointment with Dr. Boehm, who saw me a few days later. In the meantime, Dr. Smith sent him my medical records.

Dr. Boehm was a man in his mid-forties, very kind and caring. When I visited him, he had already read my medical records. Now he examined me, asked me numerous questions about my condition, and then asked me what I wanted to do. I told him that I wanted to continue with the pregnancy, but that I was afraid of it causing a stroke or a heart attack. He acknowledged the risks but said that he could monitor my progress and determine if the pregnancy was putting me in jeopardy. In the meantime, he felt that I should continue with the pregnancy. That was what I wanted to hear and I was reassured that someone would be there watching over me.

"The first thing we have to do," he said, "is remove the IUD. I'm going to be a little rough with you. If the pregnancy is good, it will hold. But if there's a problem, the baby will spontaneously abort."

He wasn't kidding. He literally yanked the thing from my body. There was some cramping and a kind of scratching pain that caused some small bleeding, but the baby stayed in place. When Dr. Boehm got the IUD out, he patted my hand and gave me a compassionate, reassuring smile. He suggested that I go home and rest. As the day progressed, I felt less and less pain and for the next two weeks, I held my breath against the fear that I might lose the baby. But no, the baby held on and each day seemed to grow stronger in my womb.

Pregnancy, as it turned out, agreed with me more than I would have ever dreamed possible. The severity of my Crohn's symptoms decreased dramatically. Throughout my pregnancy, I had significantly fewer flare-ups and I felt emotionally stable. Even the flare-ups that I did have were less severe than the ones of the past. I attributed these changes to my altered hormonal balance. Obviously, I was no longer fertile during my pregnancy; nor was I ovulating each month. Such changes in my estrogen levels might be causing the improvement in my Crohn's symptoms, I thought. In light of my improvements, Dr. Smith reduced my prednisone to 5 mg a day, the lowest it had ever been. This, of course, brought about a reduction in the side effects from the drug, which contributed even more to my feelings of health and well-being.

Meanwhile, I knew that I was going to be a mother. I felt full and rich and deeply satisfied with myself. Part of being the woman I had always dreamed of being meant being a mother, and now I was in the process of realizing that dream. Yes, I wanted more for my life—I had many ambitions—but I could not picture myself truly fulfilled unless I was a mother, too. Chip was happy, too. He was a senior in college and about to graduate that December. The idea of being a father and having a family inspired him. All of this combined to make the summer and fall of 1978 one of the best times I had experienced in a long time.

Giving Birth to a New Life

In December 1978, Chip graduated from college and got a good job in a little town near Nashville called Centerville.

Centerville was actually too small to qualify as a little town. It had one traffic light in the center of town that operated only on weekdays between 5 and 6 P.M. Otherwise, people just drove through the little hamlet as they saw fit. We started building a house not far from the center of town. Meanwhile, I continued to see Dr. Boehm, who assured me that my pregnancy was progressing normally. He told me that the baby would have to be delivered via cesarean section. He, like the other doctors, feared that if I pushed the baby out, my arteries might burst and cause severe internal bleeding. Despite my doctors assurance that a C-section would be necessary, I nonetheless took natural childbirth classes. I told myself that if there was any chance that I could give birth to my baby naturally, I wanted to do that.

In February 1979, I developed toxemia and was forced to stay in bed for the remainder of my pregnancy. As a precautionary measure, my doctors increased the dosage of prednisone that I was receiving. They seemed to get more concerned and watchful as my due date approached.

On March 14, 1979, I went into labor. Chip and I went to Vanderbilt Hospital in Nashville, about one and a half hours away. My labor was just beginning, so the doctor ordered me to stay close but walk around as much as possible. My mother had arrived from Connecticut a few days earlier along with my sister, Maritza, who was attending David Libscomb College in Nashville. We all went to a beautiful park in downtown Nashville called The Parthenon. The Parthenon is a replica of the real Parthenon in Greece. It is historic, beautiful, and the center of many musical activities in the Nashville area. As we walked and climbed The Parthenon's many steps, I would stop only to breathe through a contraction. Chip would time all the contractions with a stopwatch, and Maritza kept a written record of everything I felt. My mother was shocked that the doctors had not admitted me and shared stories of what it had been like when she had Maritza and me.

The day wore on and my labor slowly progressed. The doctors at the hospital checked me periodically and said to keep walking. They agreed that if I showed no signs of danger, I would be allowed to deliver naturally, only with the help of forceps to prevent my having to push. We spent the night at my brother and sister-in-law's duplex in Nashville. Surprisingly I slept well between the contractions. By 6 A.M., I was quite uncomfortable. By 8 A.M., I was back at the hospital. The doctors checked me, and my water broke. They were pleased with my progress and decided it was safe for me to deliver naturally.

I was changed into a hospital gown, placed on a gurney, and wheeled to a hospital room, where I was monitored for several hours. Chip remained with me in my room. My contractions were coming rapidly now and soon I was possessed by an overwhelming desire to push the baby out. "Get the nurse," I told Chip. "This is feeling different."

The nurse hurried into my room and discovered that the baby's head was crowning. "Don't push," the nurse said to me. She obviously didn't want me to give birth at that moment. She might also have been concerned about the Takayasu arteritis and the possibility that I might hemorrhage if I pushed. "I've got to push," I told her. "No, wait," she said. I tried to comply, but it was against all of my instincts.

Meanwhile, Chip rubbed my cheeks, face, arms, and legs. At the same time, he coached me in my breathing—all the things we had learned in our natural childbirth classes. The nurse must have thought that Chip's rubbing of my body was strange because she said, with some irritation, "What's he doing?"

"Oh, it's okay," I said. "It feels good. I need distraction from the pain."

Chip was white with fear. I was afraid he might pass out, but he kept rubbing me and coaching me to breathe.

The nurse said that she was going to take me down to the operating room, where I would give birth. She asked Chip if he wanted to remain behind. "No," he said. "I want to go with her."

"It's okay," I said to Chip. "You've been great. If you don't feel like you can go in there, I can make it on my own from here."

"No," he said. "I want to be with you."

I was wheeled to the operating room and Chip was escorted to a place where he could get into his scrubs. When I arrived in the operating room, I was greeted by my doctor, several nurses, and eleven medical students, all gawking at me as if I were some kind of alien being. I had been told that this was a teaching hospital and that there would be students watching me give birth. At first it seemed odd to be observed this way, but as the birth proceeded, I quickly forgot their presence.

I was immediately attached to monitoring devices and given an epidural. I was also given another shot of prednisone.

"Listen to me," I told the doctor and nurses, "I've got to push. I can't hold back."

"Don't push," a nurse said. "I'll do it for you." She got her hands under my breasts and pushed down on my diaphragm. I was amazed at how effective she was at pushing the baby for me. Meanwhile, the doctor took a pair of large metal forceps and inserted them inside of me. The sight of the forceps frightened me. They looked like a tool for some form of draconian torture. Once he had the forceps inside me, he began to pull with a force so great that I became terrified he might hurt my baby.

As all of this occurred, I began to hallucinate from the high dose of prednisone. I was seeing colors and feeling disoriented. But somehow I remained focused on what was taking place. Finally, my baby popped out. Someone told me it was a girl.

"Chip, look at her," I said to him. "Is she all right? Is she okay?"

Chip was in his own world. "Wow, she's amazing," he said.

The doctor handed the baby to Chip first, while they worked on me, and Chip held her in his arms, completely absorbed by her beauty. Meanwhile, the doctor and nurses stitched me up after the episiotomy. Chip walked over to the medical students and showed her off.

"Bring her over here, bring her over to me," I kept telling him.

Finally, my baby was in my arms. I was happier than I'd ever been in my life. I couldn't believe she was so perfect, so fine. She seemed utterly healthy to me. "Is she all right?" I asked the nurse. "Yes, she seems fine," the nurse answered. She was puffy and red, but quite content to be in my arms.

After a few minutes, the nurse took my baby away from me.

The baby needed some tests, she said. I was placed on a gurney and wheeled into a storage room and left there for several hours. All around me were linens piled high on shelves. Now the prednisone was really kicking in. I was lightheaded and seeing colors. I desperately wanted my baby; I wanted to be with my family. I wanted to celebrate the birth of my child. But instead, I lay on a gurney in some kind of storage room–wash closet. What was I doing here? I kept wondering. Why had they left me?

Finally a nurse burst in and brought me to my room. "I want to be with my baby," I told her. My baby would be with me as soon as I came down from the effects of the prednisone, she said. But it would be a full four hours before I finally got to be with my child. She had to be monitored and tested extensively because of the possible side effects of the prednisone. No one knew what her condition would be after being on a daily dose of prednisone during her entire gestation. I told Chip to stay with our daughter since I couldn't be there.

Finally, my baby was brought to me and laid in my arms. I was told that she was normal, except that she would suffer side effects from the withdrawal from the prednisone. She was already on a bottle, though I would nurse her as well for the next six months. My daughter was born on my mother's birthday, March 15, at 2 P.M., just as I had been born on my grandmother's birthday, January 8. We named her Norma Christine, after my mother, Norma, and Chip's mother, Christine. We called her Chrisi for short. My family was all in the waiting room chafing to see me and our new child. Before they entered, I got on the public address system from the phone in my room and announced to my mom, "Happy birthday! You have a granddaughter!" Later my mother told me how surprised and relieved she was by my announcement. Soon, my family all crowded into my room and celebrated the birth of our child. Finally, we had our family celebration.

Contrary to all that we had been told, our child was not handicapped in any way. She was normal and healthy. Also, I had given birth naturally, without having to undergo a C-section. And finally, I had survived the entire pregnancy and birthing process.

They were wrong on all three counts, I told myself. The realization that doctors were not infallible would prove important in the months to come.

Later, after everyone had left my room, I was finally alone with my child. I was filled with love for my little Chrisi. As I held her and examined every inch of her tiny body, I noticed that she quivered and jerked from time to time, a reaction to the withdrawal from prednisone, no doubt. I felt responsible for her suffering. Nonetheless, she was perfect, a true gift from God. All at once it hit me: I have to become strong and healthy for this little girl. She needs her mother. I have to live a long life. I have to be there as she grows up. I need my health because by daughter needs me.

3

In the Darkness, a Sudden Glimmer of Light

Looking back, I realize now that there was a kind of magic in it all. It was as if the March wind had swept in from the East, having been touched by the yellow light of the morning sun; it blew into my face and just like that my life was changed. I was a mother now. Somehow Chrisi's birth, which had occurred in a matter of hours, had enlarged my life as nothing I had ever experienced before. I had this little baby to love, to care for, and to protect. Something awesome and unfathomable had placed her life in my hands. She was so vulnerable, so trusting, so lovable. Every detail of her life—her little round face, her tiny hands, her perfect body, her small cries, her every need—aroused my maternal instinct and drew from my heart a never-ending river of love.

The thought that my daughter had been on prednisone for the previous nine months fell heavily on me. She developed scoliosis at age 11 as a consequence of the drug, but with proper attention and care, it did not progress. Her periodic quivering and sudden jerks reminded me, as well, of our mutual dependence on the prednisone. "Should I nurse her?" I had asked my pediatrician. I had been concerned that the residue of the drug in my system would taint my breast milk and cause her additional problems.

"Yes, nurse her," my doctor assured me. "It will do her more good than harm."

Like pregnancy, nursing dramatically reduced my Crohn's symptoms. I had been given another reprieve and I used it to give my attention to little Chrisi. The two of us fell into a blissful routine that was like our shared cocoon.

"Good" Southern Cookin'

Chip would be up by 6:30 A.M. and at work by 7:30. He often made his own breakfast, which usually consisted of eggs, bacon, and cheese. Omelettes were among his favorites. Chrisi and I would sleep until ten, at which point I would get up, nurse her for a while or give her a bottle, and then make myself some breakfast.

I needed as much sleep during the day as I could get because my nights were disturbed and restless, thanks again to the prednisone. I usually had trouble getting to sleep at night and would often lie awake for hours. Mostly I would read, but many nights I could not lie still and would have to get out of bed and pace the house. Sometimes I would want Chip to keep me company in the middle of the night—I needed the attention—but he couldn't be with me at those odd hours. He had to get up in the morning and work all day; he needed his sleep. At least that's what I told myself each night, but the loneliness would sometimes overwhelm me. Before Chrisi was born, I occasionally would get dressed, get into my car, and drive around town a bit. Before I went, I would tell Chip that I was going out for a drive, hoping that he would wake up and tell me to stay, that he would talk to me for a while. But he never did. "Okay," he would say to me, more asleep than awake, and instantly he would be asleep again. Chip could remain asleep through the loudest of disturbances.

After an hour or two of driving around town, I would return home, exhausted and ready for sleep. Chip would be gone when I awoke the next morning. Before he left, he would get Chrisi and put her in bed with me.

Before I could actually get out of bed, I would sit on the side of the bed and allow my feet to adjust to the feeling of the floor. In the mornings, my feet would be acutely swollen and my legs weak. I needed a moment to establish my balance and to know for sure that my feet and legs would be strong enough to let me stand up without falling over. Once I had nursed Chrisi, I would get dressed and go into the kitchen.

Breakfast was usually a quick meal of eggs and bacon, or toast, butter, and jam, or some cereal and milk. The effort of putting breakfast together often drained me of energy, however. Once I had eaten, I would clean up and then get Chrisi from her crib and bring her into my bed. We would lie there together as she slept and nursed.

I had to go to the bathroom often, thanks to the prednisone, which had made my kidneys and bladder weak. Between trips to the bathroom, I lay and rested.

Chrisi occupied most of my day. When I wasn't attending to her needs, I would lay next to her and marvel. As the months passed and she became more aware and mobile, we would lie together and play. I would keep her entertained in little ways, by playing with her toys or giving her a little tickle or just holding her while she slept.

At around 1 or 2 P.M., Chrisi would take a nap and I would have the rest of the afternoon to shower, make myself lunch, put dinner together, and then put on something nice so that I looked good when Chip got home.

Lunch consisted of poached eggs over toast, with hot chocolate, or some type of sandwich meat, such as bologna, salami, or ham with cheese. Sometimes I would make myself a peanut butter and jelly or grilled cheese sandwich. I often warmed some Campbell's soup, as well. After lunch, I would eat a bag of potato chips with dip, or some kind of sweet dessert. I liked Twinkies, or Chips A'hoy cookies, or anything with chocolate in it. Sometimes I would forgo the sandwich entirely and go directly for a piece of chocolate cake, or cookies, or a chocolate candy bar.

If I was feeling well and had the energy, I would make a chess pie, which is pretty much a staple in the South. It's made of eggs, sugar, and milk, with lots of lard in the pie crust, of course.

In the years I had lived in the South, I had become a good Southern cook, which meant that I used lots of lard and grease in nearly everything I made. Like every other woman that I knew, I kept a coffee can filled with grease under my sink. Every time I fried a food, or made eggs, bacon, sausage, or some other form of meat, I would gather up the grease in the skillet and pour it off into my coffee can. This wasn't just a little habit, but a Southern tradition.

Shortly after Chip and I were married, my mother-in-law gave me a coffee can with two inches of grease in it—a kind of starter can on my way to being a good Southern cook. She was proud to give me that grease—it was a kind of initiation into the mysteries of being a Southern wife. I was proud, as well, of all the grease that I had accumulated in my own can. I cooked everything in it, even my vegetables. And when I was finished cooking, I would pour off the grease into my coffee can for recycling.

Dinner was the focal point of every day. I very much wanted to please Chip and spent the better part of every afternoon trying to come up with something that he would really love to eat when he came home. One of his favorites, of course, was barbecue. In the North, barbecue means to cook outdoors, but in the South barbecue is a way of preparing meat, usually Boston butt, or roast rump, or some thick piece of pork.

The way you prepare good barbecue is to cook the meat all day in a crock pot that also contains barbecue sauce. As the meat cooks, you keep basting it with more barbecue sauce, either by brushing it on or by pouring it on top. You do this for about six hours, leaving the meat to cook in its juices and the sauce. When the meat has been cooked thoroughly and is very tender, you shred it with a fork so that it becomes strings of meat, thoroughly marinated with sauce. You serve it with corn bread and cole slaw. For dessert, I often made chocolate or chess pie.

Another favorite of Chip's was sour cream chicken breast, made by marinating the breast in lots of condensed cream of mushroom soup. Add salt, pepper, and spices. After the chicken sits in the soup for a few hours, remove it with the goopy soup stock still clinging and put it in a pan. At that point, you cover it with sour cream and bread crumbs, then bake it in the oven.

Occasionally, I would make spaghetti and meatballs. We typically had some form of animal food three times a day, and meat at least twice a day. Of course, one of Chip's favorites was venison, which came fresh every fall and winter, thanks to the fact that he was an avid deer hunter. Neither of us drank alcohol because his religion forbade it, which meant that we relied heavily on soda pop and milk. We drank a lot of both. We would go through at least a gallon of milk per week.

Chip usually got home between 4:45 and 5 P.M., which was when we would eat dinner. After dinner, he would play with Chrisi, I would clean up, and we would spend the evening watching television. At night, I wanted us to talk to each other. I had spent the day with the baby and wanted some adult communication. But he had been with adults all day in the pressurized world of work and wanted to escape at night in front of the television. We had opposite needs that didn't seem to want to join. In time, I grew emotionally needy—I wanted him to talk and pay attention to me, but he was quiet and introverted and wanted to talk only about work. We would retire to bed by 10:30 to get as much sleep as possible before Chrisi would wake us, first at around 1 A.M. and then again at 4 A.M., on both occasions to nurse. If we were lucky, she would fall asleep while nursing, but if she was restless, Chip would walk her for a while. The father-daughter dance would last anywhere from 15 minutes to an hour. Finally, we would all fall into a deep and much needed sleep, exhausted but content.

As spring turned to summer, we began to participate in more activities with the Church of Christ community, which scheduled weekly events. I tried to do as much as possible, but I couldn't always attend the social gatherings. Everything I did, or wanted to do, had to be planned around the condition of my intestines and my other Crohn's symptoms. If I had diarrhea, or if my headaches, nausea, or cramps were too severe, I couldn't leave my house. For this reason, I never committed myself too far in advance, no matter how badly Chip or I wanted to do something. Whenever we were invited to do something with the church, or with friends for that matter, I would always have to warn people in advance that I might have to cancel at the last minute. In time, virtually everyone in our church community and all of our friends knew about my problems. In fact, people in the church regularly prayed for me.

On the whole, I liked participating in the Church of Christ activities and I enjoyed the worship services, but I must admit that the community was composed of people who were very different from those I grew up with. The Southern Christians in our Centerville community were straightlaced and preoccupied with the accepted rules of behavior. They were bound by a strict code of manners, which made a lot of them cool and unaffectionate. Many of those rules were designed to keep men and women at some distance from each other, lest their passions arise, I suppose. Men and women were forbidden from swimming together. No one danced. Singing was often restricted to church songs. Alcohol, of course, was disapproved of, if not forbidden.

Chip fit right in, but I always felt awkward, in part because I came from a Spanish family that was more passionate and prone to outward displays of emotions. My family's parties were always full of singing, dancing, eating, and drinking. We did not do these things to excess, I should say, but we were not bound by any external code that forbade free and open self-expression. Latin blood is different, I used to tell myself, and left it at that.

Still, I enjoyed the church social gatherings whenever I could participate. And as long as I was nursing, my symptoms remained under some control. I did not experience an intense flare-up that entire summer. But in September, I weaned Chrisi, and little by little the proverbial dam started to give way. My Crohn's symptoms gradually returned. The first thing to weaken were my intestines. Diarrhea started to become common again. My cramping became worse and my headaches more frequent. Fall was coming, and as usual, my symptoms were rising. Meanwhile, a new series of difficulties emerged. My mother's tolerance of my father's behavior was coming to an end.

My Mother Finally Makes a Move

My mother called me regularly to express her misery over my father's lack of attention toward her. He had been unfaithful to her for many years, but it soon became clear that her frustration and heartache were reaching their limits. I was her confidante, her shoulder to cry on. Perhaps because I was the oldest daughter, I felt a special responsibility to help her find a way out of her dilemma. This put me in a terrible conflict. I loved both my parents, but I found myself siding with my mother and empathizing with her pain. Every week, it seemed, she would call me with a new tale of woe. My father wasn't coming home, she would say. He was humiliating her. What should she do? she would ask me.

"Leave him!" I would tell her. "Why are you there? You are with a man who shows up when he feels like it. You don't have a life there anymore." In fact, all three of her children had moved to Tennessee and were living in the Nashville area.

"How can I leave?" was her plaintive response. "This is my home. Where will I go?"

"Come here," I told her again and again. "Make a new life for yourself."

"I cannot divorce your father. We do not believe in divorce in Chile."

"Don't divorce him," I said. "Just leave him. Come here and let him decide what he wants to do."

"No, I am not ready to leave my home," my mother would say finally.

This is how the conversation went. We were like actors in a long-running play, each saying her lines with deep conviction at every performance, but always with the same unsatisfying end. The conversations left me angry at both my parents—angry at my father for his behavior, but also frustrated with my mother for staying in a bad situation. I also feared for my mother, because she was clearly becoming depressed. Her job was the only stimulus that got her out of bed each day. In fact, before I became a mother, my parents' problems had consumed me. I would lay awake at night thinking of ways in which I might be able to help them reconcile, or separate amicably, if that was the only solution. After so many years of conflict and pain, a solution didn't seem possible, at least to me. Yet, I couldn't bear them being in such misery, especially my mother, who seemed to be the more vulnerable of the two. It made me feel guilty to know that my mother was suffering, while I was happy.

After Chrisi was born, however, my feelings about my parents' problems began to change. One day at the end of the summer, my mother called and started to tell me of my father's latest episodes.

"*Mamita*, I cannot keep doing this," I said. "I have a family now. This is where my attention should be. This is what matters now. I can't keep getting involved in your problems with Dad. I have to be concerned here, in my house, with my child and husband. Unless you come up with a solution that I can help you with, I cannot keep having this conversation. You have to decide what you are going to do and then live with it."

When I said those words, I suddenly realized that they came from a place that I did not know existed within me. I had made an entirely new commitment to my child and my husband. Marriage was one thing, but motherhood was another. I had made a step in my life that was bigger than even I had realized. I felt freed from the responsibility for fixing my parents' problems.

A few days after I had said that, my mother called me.

"I'm ready to come to Nashville."

"Good," I said. "You can stay with us until you can find a place to live. It will all work out, *Mamita*," I said. "Don't worry."

By mid-September, my mother had moved to Nashville. In no time, it seemed, she had found a good job and a place to live. She had completed the crossing and obtained a divorce, and was a free woman. Little did I realize that my mother's presence would later play a major role in saving my life.

The Light Retreats

By the end of September, I realized that I would need a stronger dose of the prednisone. Up until that time, I took a very low dose—5 mg a day—but as my symptoms began to worsen, Dr. Smith increased the dose gradually until it was at 45 mg a day. As we moved deeper into the fall, it would go higher and eventually reach as much as 90 mg a day.

As before, the higher doses of prednisone brought on immediate side effects. My body swelled with added weight. I watched myself add 10, then 20, then 30 pounds. Eventually I reached 142, about 30 pounds over my normal weight.

I felt that if you pricked me with a pin, I would pop. I couldn't move without feeling that my body was in my way. My face became round, red, and swollen. At the higher doses, the drug caused my sight to become distorted. Images seemed to wiggle in the upper hemisphere of my vision. It was as if the world were split along the horizon—everything below the horizon line looked normal; everything above was slightly twisted, as if seen in a fun house mirror. Of course, my sleep was even more disturbed by the higher doses of prednisone and I was forced to take sleeping pills to get any rest at all.

The prednisone had a dramatic effect on my energy levels, as well. The drug would initially cause a rush of energy, which was eventually followed by terrible fatigue and exhaustion. Whenever I had energy, I would try to accomplish things, assuming Chrisi's needs allowed. I would run errands, go grocery shopping, cook big meals, and clean the house. But once the burst of energy waned, I would succumb to intense fatigue and eventually to depression. I came to see these bursts of energy that the prednisone gave me as my lifeline. Whatever side effects it might have caused me, the drug also made it possible for me to function.

In addition to the prednisone, I was taking Azulfidine, potassium, aspirin, a diuretic, iron, and sleeping pills. Yet, even all this medication had little effect on the disorder.

As my physical and emotional condition deteriorated, I grew increasingly needy of Chip's attention, love, and support. Unfortunately, my demands caused him to back away, which only made me more demanding and him more distant. But there was another problem that arose in the fall that separated us: hunting season arrived.

In the South, the importance of hunting, particularly deer hunting, is second only to that of religion. Some schools are closed on the first day of deer hunting season so that sons, mostly, can go with their fathers to hunt deer. So begin the rites of the season, which overtook the men of our community like a fever. Chip was no different. If he wasn't out hunting, he was planning his next hunting trip, either with his friends or by himself, often while he cleaned one of his many guns. During the season his guns tended to turn up in unexpected places. I would be hanging clothes in a closet and suddenly discover a rifle or two. Or I'd be putting away some article of clothing in his bureau and discover a handgun tucked between a couple of shirts. Several guns lay under our bed. None was loaded, however, and after a while I took them all for granted.

Within the hunting season are several miniseasons. Weeks are set aside for hunting wild turkey, dove, pheasant, quail, duck, and many other animals. There are also miniseasons for the different ways to hunt deer—with a bow, for example, or a shotgun. This allows hunters the opportunity to take more than one deer per year, if they are lucky enough to get one at all. Most do and Chip was a good hunter, which meant that each year we had a large supply of venison.

I didn't know much about hunting and never had the desire to learn how to hunt, either. But if this was something that we could do together, I was willing to give it a try. One day, Chip took me out to the woods to teach me how to fire a rifle. Every time I pulled the trigger I had to close my eyes and the rifle would jump off my shoulder. Eventually he became exasperated and said, "You know what? Don't hunt."

I couldn't blame him. Chip loved to hunt. Actually, it was more than love. It was an almost mystical pursuit of the kill, and the skill needed to do it well. Hunting is an act that connects men to their primitive instincts and, at the same time, to the beauty and mystery of nature. This was the way Chip experienced a reunion with nature: to be in the forest looking for animals that are beautiful, elusive, and in many ways utterly inscrutable. The otherworldliness of the forest, with its almost cathedral-like recesses, and the mysterious behavior of the animals that live within it, make the entire experience almost magical. For the hunters, the pursuit of the animals and the exploration of their habitats are a kind of communion with nature.

Anyone who could not understand or fully participate in that communion was excluded from the ritual. Such a person was also excluded from the bond hunters experience with each other. Chip and his hunting friends knew that bond. Because I wasn't able to shoot a rifle properly or hunt, I was outside that unique circle.

If anyone had asked me, I would have said that I felt the beauty and wonder of nature, too, but I never felt the need to kill something to fully enjoy it. I did not say such things to Chip, of course. He wouldn't understand my feelings. The separation that existed between us would have been even greater if he had believed that I did not understand his.

I gave him as much freedom to enjoy hunting as I could. That was not always easy, however. He and his friends were constantly getting together to plan hunting trips—where and when they would hunt. Once the trips were planned, they would go off on their expeditions, usually for a full day or a weekend. Sometimes it would be longer. Hunting season lasted from September till January.

By October, my symptoms would be raging. I would have regular pounding headaches, bouts of diarrhea, cramps, and nausea. Occasionally, when a flare-up became more intense, I would experience bloody stools. Invariably, my flare-ups occurred when Chip had a hunting trip planned. Before Chip would leave, he would ask me if I was going to be all right. "Yes," I would tell him, but my heart wasn't in it.

"Why do you always get sick when I go hunting?" he would ask me.

"I don't know," I said. At that point, both of us felt guilty and I had to let him go. Still, my symptoms flared even on the days and weekends that he didn't go hunting.

Once he was gone, I was left alone with the baby and my own physical problems and emotional conflicts. My loneliness and feelings of isolation were acute. I resented him for not being home to help me, but at the same time I knew that he had every right to go hunting with his friends. I should support him, I told myself. He didn't do anything to deserve a sick wife. I knew that he was coping with my problems as best he could. Part of me was grateful to him for sticking with me through all my sickness. On the other hand, part of me resented him for his lack of attention and for leaving me to take care of the baby and my illness alone.

As we entered November, my symptoms showed no sign of abating. The suffering alone made me intensely miserable and depressed. I had dark circles under my eyes from lack of sleep. I felt distraught, pessimistic about the future, and critical of everything around me. I felt that I might be losing control of my life. All these dark emotions showed on my face.

It was late that month that my doctor suggested that I take a more powerful drug—methotrexate, he called it. Dr. Smith followed that recommendation with the statement that I would very likely require the first of many surgeries to remove the diseased parts of my small intestine, as well. We'd watch it for another month or so, he said, but if things did not get any better, he would schedule me for surgery in late January of the new year. The thought of a more intense drug and surgery terrified me. I knew that once I started down that road, it was just a matter of time before I would need an ileostomy and be forced to wear a bag on my side. The thought of such a fate made me even more desperate to find an answer.

A Sliver of Light

Throughout that fall, I explored various natural methods for treating my Crohn's disease. I regularly went to the health food store to buy vitamins, herbs, and herbal teas. Someone who worked there once told me that slippery elm was good for the intestines so I took that, along with vitamin C and an array of minerals. Nothing affected my illness, but I continued to look for answers.

Fortunately, I was not alone in my search. My father, mother, grandmother, and aunts were all passionately searching for answers, as well. Each of them would call me with the new bits of information that they discovered. Nothing proved helpful, but their love and support were medicine enough for me.

And then, in mid-December, something happened that changed my life. My father called, almost breathless, and told me that he had information for me that was going to help me. He had spoken to one of his clients, someone to whom he had sold insurance whose eleven-year-old daughter had Takayasu's arteritis. This woman's daughter was practicing a strange diet that was helping her, my father said. The diet was called macrobiotics.

"*Mi hijita,*" my little daughter, he said. "You are going to have to eat a lot of weird foods, like seaweed and this thing called miso, but this is going to work. I know it. This makes sense. Your problem is in the intestines and that's where the food goes. I'll do it with you. You're going to get better. You'll see."

I was taken aback by his enthusiasm. I could picture my father on the other end of the phone—his strong, handsome, Latin face; and that trim little mustache dancing as he spoke. My father is a strong man who is softened by his love and enthusiasm for life. Now, his desire that I be healthy and happy was brimming over in every word that he spoke.

"All right," I said, more than a little hesitant. I didn't know what to say. He was so emotional, so convinced that he had found the answer to my problems.

He continued: "I'm going to find the person who you should talk to for more information about macrobiotics. I will call you back. Don't worry. This is going to work. I know it."

The following day, my father called back. "The person you should call is named Bill Spear," my father said. "He is a teacher of macrobiotics. He's in Middletown, Connecticut. He can help you. You will have to call him and arrange an appointment to see him." He then gave me Bill Spear's number.

I looked at the number and for a moment I hesitated. This is going to be another doctor, or nutritionist—whatever—who is going to tell me the same old, tired things that I had already heard dozens of times before. Nothing had helped me to this point. I was taking powerful drugs and about to try even stronger medication. Even so, my doctor had little faith that the drug therapy would help me, which meant that I would undergo surgery in a month's time. What could this man offer me that I was not already doing? I wondered. Part of me was urging caution. I didn't want to get my hopes up and then be disappointed. My emotional state was fragile. I wanted so desperately to be well, but I was terrified of how a disappointment might affect me. What should I do? Suddenly, the memory of my father's enthusiasm cut through my reverie. I picked up the phone and dialed the number.

When Bill Spear answered, I introduced myself and then proceeded to explain that I had Takayasu arteritis and Crohn's disease. "Do you know anything about Takayasu arteritis?" I asked him. He had heard of it, he said. "Do you know anything about Crohn's disease?" I asked. Yes, he told me. He had worked with people with the disorder.

He asked me to describe my symptoms. After I had finished, he said something very peculiar that struck me deeply.

"The two conditions are related," he said.

As soon as he'd said those words, my entire life condition elevated. I had had the same feeling, I thought to myself. When I had first been diagnosed with Crohn's disease in Virginia, the doctor had showed me x-rays of both the arteries in my neck, which were affected by the Takayasu disease, and my intestines, which were affected by the Crohn's. They looked very much alike. At the time, I pointed this out to my doctor and said, "These two conditions look very similar. Is it possible that they are related in some way?"

"No," the Virginia doctor had assured me—not without a little condescension. "They're very different diseases," he said. "One is a blood disease and the other is an intestinal disease."

Now, without even seeing me, Bill Spear was telling me something that deep down I had suspected all along. Yes, I thought to myself. These two illnesses are somehow related.

"Can macrobiotics help me?" I asked.

"Yes," he said. "But you will have to start immediately."

"I'm supposed to start a new round of drugs next month and then have part of my intestines removed," I told him.

"If you want to avoid the surgery, you will have to start right away and you will have to be very strict on the diet and lifestyle that I recommend for you."

"How will this diet help me?" I asked.

"Go out and buy the book *Sugar Blues* by William Dufty. That will explain the effects of sugar and processed foods on your intestines. It will also explain a lot about how a change in your diet can help reverse your condition. In the meantime, write a short history of your health issues and send it to me."

With that, we set up an appointment and I made arrangements to fly to Connecticut to see Bill Spear.

I called my father back and told him the news. He was elated. "I will go with you," he assured me. "I'll help you. We'll do the diet together."

When Chip got home, I told him everything that had happened. "You know, this may be something worthwhile," I said to Chip.

"Well, don't get your hopes up," he answered.

Neither of us said anything for a minute. All of a sudden, Chip realized the potential consequences of what I had been saying.

"Good night alive, Ginny," he said. "You're going to have to eat hippy food—tofu!"

4

The Strange and Miraculous World of Macrobiotics

He didn't look like a hippy.

That was my first thought upon being introduced to Bill Spear, the macrobiotic counselor whom my father had found and believed could help me. He was young—thirty years old, as it turned out—and nice looking. Clean cut, dark eyes, dark hair, and healthy looking. He didn't have a doctor's air about him, which wasn't a bad thing, as far as I was concerned. I had seen more than my share of doctors, without much relief.

Bill Spear's office was in Middletown, Connecticut, about an hour north of Stamford. As he drove us there, my father exhibited the same outward excitement about macrobiotics that he had conveyed on the telephone two weeks before. "I think this is going to help you," he said again. "I think this is it."

My parents had suffered through so many health crises with me that none of us could keep track of them now. On the way to Bill Spear's office, my father recalled some of those dark times. "I remember the first time you got sick at school," he said. "You had such terrible pain and cramps that the school sent you home," my father recalled. "That night, you blacked out from the pain and we had to take you to the emergency room at the hospital. That was the beginning. After that, so many trips to the hospital . . . ." He shook his head in wonder at all that I had been through—all that *we* had been through.

You don't realize how much parents suffer with a sick child until after you are a parent yourself. Only then do you know the pain and powerlessness that parents feel when they have to watch their child go through illness, but can do nothing to help. Now that I had little Chrisi, I realized all the more how much hardship my father and mother had suffered with me. I didn't want to go through anything like that with my daughter.

Now, as my father, Bill Spear, and I shook hands and took our respective chairs, I was glad my dad was with me. I didn't know what to expect, but I was more cautious than optimistic.

Spear gave me some paperwork to fill out that requested some basic information about the reason I had come to see him. When I was finished, he asked us if my father was going to stay and if that was all right with me. Yes, to both questions, I said.

"That's good," he said. "It's essential that you have family support."

My father announced that he was going to do this with me. "That's great," was Spear's response.

"May I look at your hands?" he asked.

"Of course," I said.

He then proceeded to do the strangest examination of me that I had ever experienced. He looked closely at my hands, arms, and feet. He then examined my eyes and my face very thoroughly. As he did, he asked me questions or made an occasional comment.

"You like milk and you ate a lot of chicken growing up," he said, as he conducted his examination.

I laughed. "Yes, we were raised on a chicken farm in Chile."

"You've eaten a lot of sugar, too," he said with a little laugh. I gave a little embarrassed laugh, too.

"When you wake up at night at around two A.M., is it because you have to go to the bathroom or because you're awakened by a noise or pain?"

"I usually have to go to the bathroom," I said. But to myself, I asked, How does he know I have to get up at 2 A.M.?

"The pain you feel in your intestines—is it located in one

place or does it radiate throughout your intestinal tract?" he asked me.

"It radiates through my abdomen."

"I see," he said, more to himself than to me. "By the way, what did you think about *Sugar Blues?*"

William Dufty's book was an exposé on the impact of sugar on history, economies, and health. He shows how sugar was a highly expensive luxury item right up through the 1800s—whiskey was cheaper, Dufty points out—and how its cost prevented the stuff from being used widely by anyone at the time, especially children. The cost of sugar, Dufty points out, acted as a kind of protection from the stuff. In some traditional cultures, the physicians saw sugar as a powerful drug and used it medicinally in tiny portions. But at the turn of the century, sugar became much more widely accessible until it was available to anyone, including children. It was at that point that people began to be addicted. And with that addiction came a whole new set of illnesses. Dufty quotes a New Jersey dentist who, in 1912, took note of these changes.

"Modern manufacturing of sugar has brought about entirely new diseases," the dentist, a Dr. Robert Boesler, stated. "The sugar of commerce is nothing else but concentrated crystallized acid. If, in former times sugar was so costly and that only the wealthy could afford to use it, it was, from the national economic standpoint, of no consequence. But today, when, because of its low cost, sugar has caused a degeneration of the people, it is time to insist on a general enlightenment. The loss of energy through the consumption of sugar in the last century can never be made good, as it has left a mark on the race. Alcohol has been used for thousands of years and has never caused the degeneration of a whole race. Alcohol does not contain destructive acids."

Dufty goes on to document how that "crystallized acid" precipitates a series of biochemical crises that affects the intestines, kidneys, pancreas, adrenal glands, and brain. Eventually, it breaks down the body and distorts the mind. He quotes endocrinologist John W. Tintera as saying, "It is quite possible to improve your disposition, increase your efficiency, and change your personality for the better. The way to do it is to avoid cane and beet sugar in all forms and guises." Dufty went on to document how sugar produces diabetes, helps to raise cancer rates, brings about an epidemic of hypoglycemia, and destroys digestion. The book made me wonder just how much damage I had done to myself. Certainly my intestines felt as if they had been awash in acid for most of my life.

"The book made so much sense to me," I told Bill Spear. "I never knew sugar was causing all those problems."

"That's one of the things you're going to learn," Bill Spear said to me. "How sugar is affecting your body."

He completed his examination of me and resumed his chair. "What do you want to do after you are well?" he asked me.

The question caught me off guard. He hadn't told me anything as yet about the macrobiotic diet or how it might help me.

"I'm going to be happy," I said with a little laugh.

"No, no," he said. "Be specific. What does happiness look like to you? What image does it bring up? What do you see yourself doing after all the pain and self-consuming symptoms are gone?"

I took a minute to think about that. "I picture myself one day riding my bike with my daughter," I said. For a moment, my voice stammered as a rush of emotion filled my throat. "I want to watch my daughter grow up."

"Your daughter is going to be how old then?" he asked.

"About six or seven," I said.

"Good. You hold on to that image, especially through the next few months, because they're going to be difficult. Are you religious people? Do you have a faith that you practice?"

My father answered. "Of course we believe in God. We pray a lot."

"Okay," Bill Spear said. "Then you pray a lot that this works for you. And, have the faith that it will."

An Alternate World of Food and Healing

With that, he launched into his explanation of what was causing my disease and how macrobiotics was going to help me get well. He said that meat, chicken, and dairy products such as milk and cheese are all rich in protein and fat. Once in the body, protein is converted into uric acid, which courses through the blood and acts on sensitive tissues, including the kidneys and digestive tract. High uric acid levels also cause the loss of minerals throughout the body, including from the bones. At the same time, the liver reacts to the presence of high-fat foods by secreting high levels of bile acids, which the body uses to break down fat so that it can be eliminated through the intestines. However, as the bile acid levels increase, they accumulate within the intestines and act upon the very sensitive intestinal tissues, eating away at them and creating ulcers, sores, and exposed wounds. Other acidic foods, such as sugar, tomatoes, eggplant, potatoes, and tropical fruits, add to the acid burden of the digestive tract. Together, these foods create the very conditions that give rise to Crohn's disease.

The body attempts to rid itself of the acidity and the toxins in these foods through natural processes, such as bowel movements, urination, and exhalation. The skin eliminates toxins, as well, by sweating, blemishes, and other skin discharges. But when the poisons become overwhelming, the body has to use more drastic measures to rid itself of them. One of the ways it does that is diarrhea.

"But you just named all the foods that I eat," I said. "What can I eat if not those foods?"

"There is a whole group of foods that will help your body heal," he said. He then named some of the foods: whole grains such as brown rice, barley, millet, corn, wheat, and oats; a wide variety of fresh vegetables such as collard, kale, mustard greens, broccoli, squash, carrots, and other roots; beans such as azuki, lentils, and pinto beans; and sea vegetables such as arame, hiziki, and nori.

As he ran off this list, which was quite extensive, the thought hit me that he didn't understand Crohn's disease at all. He doesn't realize that I can't eat those foods, I thought.

"Grains, vegetables, beans—those are the foods that the doctors tell me to stay away from," I said. "And I know that when I eat those foods, they drive me straight to the bathroom."

Spear's composure did not waver. "I understand," he said. "We have to reteach your body to be able to eat these foods. These are the foods that are going to help your body heal, but we have to prepare them so that your body can accept and digest them." He then explained that I would have to cook these foods with a lot of water to make them very moist and soft. My foods would have to be almost the consistency of baby foods.

He then went into great length about the importance of chewing.

"Chewing not only breaks down the food," he said, "but alkalizes it. Food that is slightly alkaline will balance and soothe your acidic digestive tract. I will give you other foods that will alkalize your digestive system even more.

"Chewing also causes the food to be infused with the enzyme amylase, which starts the breakdown and digestion of carbohydrate. Digestion begins in the mouth. By chewing, you take a great deal of stress off your digestive tract. Chewing makes digestion easier."

I was starting to understand. What he said made sense to me. Whenever I had a flare-up and was hospitalized, the doctors always gave me soft foods such as Jell-O, pudding, milk, and soft-boiled eggs. But as Spear explained it, the hospital foods were acid-producing and difficult to digest, as were most of the other foods on my every-day diet. I always believed that food had something to do with the cause of my disease. I just never understood what.

He also allayed my fears about the fibrous nature of the macrobiotic foods. By making them moist and soft, these foods would be easier to digest.

"The food should be moist, sometimes even a bit watery," he said. "Also, I'd like you to eat miso soup twice a day, once in the morning with your breakfast and a second time at dinner." He proceeded to describe miso as a fermented soybean paste that is rich in beneficial bacteria and digestive enzymes. Miso is aged in sea salt, which makes it highly alkalizing to the blood and to the entire digestive tract. Miso, I would learn, is loaded with immune-boosting and cancer-fighting properties. "Miso will help to heal your intestines," Bill Spear said.

"I'd also like you to drink a tea called ume-sho-kuzu," he told me. He then proceeded to give me a recipe filled with foreign-sounding foods. The tea is made by dissolving kuzu in cold water. Kuzu is a white, rock-like powder that is derived from the root of the kudzu plant. The water is brought to a boil. A small Japanese pickled plum, called an umeboshi plum, is placed in the water before it is boiled and then cooked as the water comes to a boil. The dissolved kuzu is added to the water and then stirred. (Precise instructions for making kuzu tea can be found in Chapter 12.) Gradually, the tea thickens into a Jell-O-like consistency. Once it has become viscous, a couple of drops of traditionally made shoyu, or soy sauce, is mixed into the water. You drink the thick liquid and eat the plum.

Kuzu is extremely healing to the intestines, Bill said. Because the tea is made with the pickled plum and shoyu, it is also extremely alkalizing, which Spear said would promote the healing of my digestive tract. He wanted me to drink the ume-sho-kuzu three times a day.

"Your body is going to go through a lot of changes," he said. "You're going to start detoxifying, or discharging the poisons, which may cause some symptoms. You may have some diarrhea or mucous discharge. Different people eliminate in different ways. But this elimination is part of the healing process. You're going to purge your system of a lot of the poisons that are now creating your Crohn's disease and Takayasu arteritis."

"But I'm already having those symptoms," I said.

"Yes, but when you adopt macrobiotics, the elimination you experience will be much less severe, much more controlled. It won't bring about the kind of crisis that you have gone through up till now."

At that point, he asked me a very strange question: "Do you have a gas or electric stove?"

"An electric stove," I said. "Why?"

"You're going to need a gas stove," Bill Spear said. "As you learn more about macrobiotics, you'll understand that food is not just nutrition, but energy. The quality of that energy helps determine whether or not we heal. That's why the preparation of the food is so important, because the way we wash and cut the food, the quality of the cookware, the orderliness of the kitchen and home, and even the respect we give the food—all of these affect the healing power of the food. A gas range that gives a good clean fire infuses the food with a deep and powerful healing energy." Electric cooking, he said, infuses the food with a diffuse, superficial, and chaotic energy, which becomes part of the food and, when eaten, part of our bodies. That chaotic energy prevents deep healing. "Besides," he said, "you will find that cooking food on a gas range will make it much more delicious than cooking on an electric stove. Of course, the flavor of the food reflects its quality. Weak and poorly prepared food does not taste as good as well-prepared food that's full of vital energy."

"What about the drugs I'm taking?" I asked. "Will I ever be able to get off them?"

"Yes," Bill Spear said. "As your doctor sees that your condition is improving, he will naturally start reducing the medications little by little until you are weaned from them entirely. But for the time being, we must allow your system to heal. So we're not going to worry about the drugs now."

"How long will it take before I start to feel better?" I asked.

"There will be a lot of changes over the next few weeks," Bill Spear said. "You'll begin to experience the effects of the food and you'll start to see improvements. But you should see very significant improvement over the next four months, which is how long it will take to change your cells dramatically. New cells will be created from the nutrients provided by the foods that you will be eating."

He looked at me for a long moment and then said, "You can turn this around. But if you want to avoid the new drugs and the surgery, you will have to start right away and you've got to follow the diet without going back to any of the old foods. One day, you will appreciate and be thankful for this experience. The illness is your teacher."

I gave a confused nod and thought, "Appreciate my disease? This guy just doesn't realize all I've been through!"

Bill then gave me several sheets of paper that described the diet in extensive detail. They not only detailed what to eat, but what not to eat. After he went over the sheets with the dietary recommendations, the consultation was over. We all shook hands and he encouraged me to call him whenever I had any questions.

Before leaving, I bought two books: *The Book of Macrobiotics* by Michio Kushi and *Introducing Macrobiotic Cooking* by Wendy Esko and Aveline Kushi.

When my father and I were back in the car, we were both excited and overwhelmed. But as usual, my father's indomitable spirit transcended all the questions we had.

"This makes sense, Ginny," my father said. "We did this in Chile. In Chile, the food is unprocessed; it's whole foods. Here, it's all processed. And you weren't sick in Chile. I know this is right. We can do this. And we'll all do this with you." He gave me that beautiful, intimate smile of his, which was full of love. My father had a way of making himself available in times of crisis. I felt the closest to him when I was ill because I had his full attention.

But Can I Do It?

In a way, my father was attempting to allay the obvious fears that we both felt at that moment, most of which coalesced around a single question: How am I going to do this? When I got out of the consultation, my head was swimming. How will I ever learn how to prepare all these foreign foods? Will I be able to stick to the diet that Bill Spear described? He made it clear that I couldn't deviate from his guidelines. But would I be able to stick to such a strict diet without succumbing to my cravings and temptations? And how would Chip react to all of this? He won't eat this way. I'm going to have to cook two sets of meals every day, one for Chip and another for me.

When we got to my father's house, I immediately called Chip and told him about my experience with Bill Spear. Contrary to all that I had feared, Chip was extremely supportive.

"I'll eat whatever you have to eat," he said. "If this is what you have to do, I'll do it, too. And if I want real food, I'll just go out and get it."

His words opened my heart and lifted a barrier between me and macrobiotics that had been there just a few minutes before. Maybe I could do this, I told myself. Maybe, if I just apply myself and try really hard, I can do it.

That night, I began reading the two books I had purchased. Reading *The Book of Macrobiotics* was like being dropped into Wonderland—or was it the reverse? Was I actually escaping Wonderland? Had I been living in some corrupt and thoroughly insane world in which all the foods that I had been taught to believe were good for me were actually making me sick? Was that possible? How could that be? I kept asking myself. Everyone ate this way. How could everyone that I knew be wrong? How could the entire country and most of the Western World eat food that was poison—indeed, that was killing most of us—while at the same time believing that our food was healthy and delicious? The macrobiotic viewpoint turned the entire world on its head.

As if all of that were not enough, there were other equally troubling thoughts that perplexed me. How was it possible for these macrobiotic people, who were not medically trained, to have an answer to illnesses that baffled the greatest minds in medicine? And if they did have answers, why weren't doctors beating paths to the doors of macrobiotic counselors such as Bill Spear?

Michio Kushi's book begins with an introduction to the underlying philosophy of macrobiotics, a philosophy he refers to as the order of the universe. The underlying principle of the order of the universe is the ancient understanding of yin and yang. Yin and yang are opposite and complementary forces that give rise to and shape all natural phenomena, Kushi writes. Yin is the force that causes expansion, diffusion, and dispersion. Yang is the force that creates contraction, fusion, and assimilation. Yin makes things more inactive, more passive, cooler, wetter, and softer. Yang makes things more active, more aggressive, hotter, drier, and harder. Yin is associated with the feminine, the moon, and nighttime; yang with more masculine characteristics, the sun, and daytime. When applied to the human body, the yin part of the body is the exterior and upper region, above the diaphragm. This includes the upper extremities, skin, upper part of the lungs, throat, face, and central nervous system, including the brain. The yang parts of the body are those that are deep within and below the diaphragm, such as the lower part of the lungs, liver, lower intestinal tract, reproductive organs, and legs. The heart is considered a yang organ, as well.

Individual foods and their effects could be understood in terms of yin and yang. Fruit, fruit juice, processed foods, sugar, and alcohol are all yin, which means they create expansion and diffusion. The more a person eats these foods, the more expansive and dispersing influences he takes into his body. Those influences eventually cause swelling, overweight, the breakdown or decay of tissues, and various kinds of disorders, including skin discharges, nervous system disorders, overweight, diabetes, and Crohn's disease. Yang foods, such as salt, red meat, eggs, chicken, hard cheese, and fish all create contraction, tightness, and assimilation. If these foods dominate the diet, they give rise to yang diseases, such as coronary heart disease, colon and prostate cancer, and other solid tumors.

Whole grains, such as brown rice, barley, millet, and whole wheat, are balanced, but slightly yang. This means that they create mild contraction and activity. Indeed, they are energy foods, rich in complex carbohydrates. Beans are slightly yin on the yin-yang spectrum. The bigger the bean, the more yin it is. Vegetables that grow aboveground, such as leafy greens and broccoli, are more yin than beans; those plants that grow belowground, such as carrots, parsnips, and burdock, are more yang than the aboveground vegetables. Fruit is more yin than vegetables; fruit juice more yin than fruit; processed foods more yin than fruit juice; and refined sugar even more yin. At the farthest extreme of yin are most of the recreational drugs, which are the most refined and most expansive substances consumed by people.

All the environmental influences that affect our lives can be seen in terms of yin and yang, as well. Yin influences create relaxation and rest; yang influences create contraction, activity, and speed. A warm bath, for example, is said to be yin; stress, which creates physical contraction or tension, is yang.

Macrobiotic philosophy maintains that yin and yang are constantly attracting each other and attempting to make balance. People who eat foods that have extremely contracting influences, such as salt, red meat, eggs, and hard cheeses, are therefore naturally attracted to sugar and alcohol. If the yang influences become extreme enough, the person will be attracted to the most extreme form of yin, which is drugs. While yin and yang are always attracting each other and making balance, extremes of each nonetheless create side effects. Eating an excess of animal foods creates illness, just as eating excesses of sugar, processed foods, and alcohol do.

The macrobiotic approach encourages people to eat foods that are found more in the center of the yin-yang spectrum. These foods are the most balanced, thus creating balance within the body. They also promote health by providing optimal nutrition and abundant energy while containing the fewest toxins such as fat, cholesterol, and artificial ingredients. According to macrobiotic philosophy, they are the foods humans were designed to eat.

Kushi goes to great lengths in his *Book of Macrobiotics* to show that humans evolved on a diet made up largely of whole grains, beans, fresh vegetables, sea vegetables, fish, and fruit. Plant foods were the most abundantly available to our ancestors and thus shaped our biological, psychological, and spiritual evolution.

Kushi points to the long digestive tracts of humans, more characteristic of herbivores than carnivores. Long digestive tracts are needed to break down and assimilate nutrients from plant foods. Carnivores, or meat eaters, have much shorter digestive tracts to protect them from the rancidity and disease that occur when meat remains in the intestines for too long. Humans have 32 teeth, Kushi writes, 20 of which are molars, 8 incisors, and only 4 canine teeth. Molars are designed for grinding grain, incisors for biting off vegetables, and canines for chewing flesh. This ratio—4 to 2 to 1—reveals that our diets should be composed of at least 6 parts plant food for every 1 part animal food. Our saliva is alkaline, not acidic, as is the saliva of carnivores.

Our evolution reveals the secrets to our health, Kushi maintains. As long as we follow the diet we are designed to eat, we can sustain our health, psychological happiness, and spiritual development. If we deviate from our principle foods, primarily grains and vegetables, we suffer illness, impaired judgment, and premature death.

Grain was the foundation of every culture and every civilization. Indeed, grains and vegetables, he maintains, are the keys to understanding health, evolution, and human destiny.

Macrobiotics does not restrict its understanding of food solely to the philosophy of yin and yang. It emphasizes the importance of nutrition, optimal nutrient intake, and the elimination of toxins—such as fat, cholesterol, artificial ingredients, and sugar—from the diet. It is essential, Kushi maintains, to understand food from both the energetic perspective (or yin-yang philosophy) and the nutritional perspective to create a balanced and healthful diet.

There are days that you look back upon as turning points in your life. This was one of those days for me. My consultation with Bill Spear and my brief reading of these books somehow changed me fundamentally. I didn't understand all of what I had read, but in some magical and unexpected way, it all moved me. When I finally closed *The Book of Macrobiotics* that night, I realized that I would never see the world in the same way again. What had I stumbled upon? I wondered.

Chrisi and I flew back to Tennessee, where my life would take a new direction.

5

Deeper into the Mystery

I decided to begin the macrobiotic diet on January 8, 1980, my twenty-fourth birthday. This was my birthday present to myself, I said. What better day to begin my new life?

The day before I started the macrobiotic diet, I cleaned out most of my old foods from my pantry and refrigerator. I left a stash of things for Chip—eggs, bacon, various meats, and even some milk—but those things were off-limits to me now. The rest of the food I bagged up and brought to our church, where it would be handed out to the needy. I restocked my shelves with the macrobiotic staples: brown rice, barley, millet, oats, a variety of beans, seaweeds, a couple of different types of tea, kuzu, miso, shoyu, and a dark liquid similar to shoyu called tamari. I bought lots of leafy green vegetables, broccoli, carrots, onions, and a long white radish called daikon.

I also purchased a three-burner camping stove that I placed on top of my electric range. Below the range, in one of my lower cabinets, I kept a small propane tank that supplied the gas. Everything was in place, I told myself. Now the rest was up to me.

That night, Chip and I went out to a restaurant, where I ordered the biggest piece of prime rib that I could handle. I also had a baked potato, salad, and wine. I topped off the meal with a big dessert. If this was goodbye to all of that, then I wanted my final meal to be memorable. I wanted it to be the epitome of my former life.

At dinner, I confided to Chip how much pressure I felt about starting macrobiotics.

"This is my last chance, Chip," I told him. "It makes sense to me. I've got to give my all to this. I'm afraid that if I don't do it right, I'll never get well." Chip encouraged me to adopt the macrobiotic diet and assured me that I had the strength to make it work for me.

But could I do it? I kept asking myself. Could I change myself? Did I have what it would take to make macrobiotics the foundation of my new life? That night, after we returned home from the restaurant and Chip got into bed, I stayed up and prayed for hours for God to give me the discipline and strength to make macrobiotics work for me. "Don't let me fail, God," I kept saying. "This is an answer from you. Give me the strength to do it. Don't let me mess this up." My prayers turned into tears, which turned into more prayers and more tears, until finally I was more exhausted than afraid. "It's up to you, God," I finally said. "I can't do this alone." The image of me riding a bicycle with my six-year-old daughter suddenly appeared before my mind's eye. "I've got to hold on to that image," I told myself. "I've got to do this for Chrisi, for Chip, and for me."

Before I went to bed, I poured some brown rice into a bowl and added water to soak it overnight. Chip and I had agreed that he would come home for lunch the next day and I would have a macrobiotic meal waiting for him. The menu for that meal would consist of brown rice, vegetables stir-fried in a little sesame oil, and miso soup with vegetables and wakame seaweed. With that I went to bed.

I awoke the next morning with great excitement for the challenge I was about to undertake. I got out of bed with my usual caution, allowing my feet to feel the floor for a few minutes and testing the strength of my ankles. I had had a restless night's sleep due to my indulgent meal, but I awoke that morning optimistic and excited to start my new life.

Outside, the sun sent a bright, crystal-clear light upon the earth and the sky was a faraway blue. Was it an omen? I didn't know, but it was always nice to have beautiful weather on my birthday. Nature was smiling upon me, perhaps.

I made a simple breakfast of oatmeal and some kukicha twig tea, a Japanese tea that is made by boiling water and tea twigs. The oatmeal was plain, but not bad. The tea was mild but settling. We were off to a good start, I thought.

After I had finished breakfast and cleaned up, I set about making my first real macrobiotic meal. I took out the bag of seaweed and poured it into a bowl of water. My cookbook, *Introducing Macrobiotic Cooking*, said that the seaweed should be soaked before it was used in soup or boiled. By soaking the seaweed and then pouring off the water, I could eliminate some of the excess sodium. I let the seaweed sit in the water and started cutting the vegetables that I would use in my stir-fry. With the vegetables cut, I drained the rice and put it into my new pressure cooker. I added a pinch of sea salt and several cups of fresh water. I then fastened the lid onto the pot and lit the flame. Now I turned my attention to the vegetables. I brushed the pan with sesame oil, added the vegetables and some water, and turned on the flame.

With that I turned my attention to the bowl containing the seaweed. Oh my gosh, I thought. What happened? The water had caused the seaweed to swell beyond anything that I had expected. It was now crawling over the sides of the bowl and making its way in all directions on my counter. "That was a small package of seaweed!" I said out loud. "What's going on?" What had appeared to me as a small quantity of seaweed had turned into enough food to feed a Japanese village, it seemed.

Meanwhile, the pressure cooker began hissing wildly. I ran over to the pot and turned down the flame. How long do I cook the rice over a low flame? I wondered again. I checked the book. Okay, 40 to 45 minutes.

I went back to the seaweed, gathered it up off the counter, poured off the soaking water, and placed the whole mess into a large pot. I filled the pot with water and placed it on one of the burners. I turned on the flame and let the seaweed start cooking.

Then I went back to cutting the broccoli that I would use in the miso soup.

"Okay, you're doing fine," I told myself. "Just keep an eye on things."

Was that the smell of something burning? I asked myself. Ahhh! The rice! The flame is too high! I turned it down even lower. I hope it wasn't burning for too long. Now what was I doing? Oh, the vegetables. I cut more broccoli and poured the treetops into the pot that contained the water and seaweed. The seaweed had grown even more and was now taking up the entire pot. It swam around in the water like slimy green ribbons. There was hardly any room in the pot for the broccoli. What's going on in there? The crackle of my stir-fried vegetables called my attention back to the frying pan. Okay, turn down the flame. You're burning the vegetables. No, I'm just browning the vegetables. They'll taste better that way.

How's the rice doing? The regulator on the pressure cooker issued a low hiss.

Seems okay, I told myself. How's the soup? Gosh, what is that smell? I looked into the pot of soup and then quickly turned away. It's the seaweed! It smells awful. How am I going to eat that stuff?

Suddenly, my attention was called to the frying pan. Turn off the vegetables! You're burning them! After I turned off the flame, I noticed that the vegetables were drier than I wanted them to be.

How long has the rice been on? I didn't check the time when I turned down the flame. Let's see, I'm supposed to let the rice cook in the pressure cooker for 40 to 45 minutes. How much time has passed? Fifteen minutes, I think. Close enough.

How long do I have to cook the seaweed again? Twenty minutes, according to the book. How's the broccoli doing in there? Seems fine. Ugh, that smell is going to knock me out.

I got out my little container of miso and prepared to add a big wooden spoonful to the soup. Don't forget, I told myself. You have to turn off the flame before you add the miso to the soup. I had read that miso should not be boiled because it contains digestive enzymes and friendly bacteria that would be destroyed if boiled. I turned off the flame and then added the miso paste to the soup and stirred. The "aroma" from the soup filled the house. I turned my head away as I stirred, occasionally looking into the soup to determine if the miso was dissolving. When the soup appeared to have an even consistency, I let it sit on the stove and then spooned the stir-fried vegetables into a serving bowl. The vegetables were clearly burned. Should I add anything to give them flavor? I wondered. No, I have to learn to enjoy the flavor of the vegetables themselves. I tasted a sliced carrot. Nothing. No taste at all.

Dejected, I sat down at the kitchen table and waited for the rice to finish cooking. Don't worry, I told myself. It's your first time cooking a macrobiotic meal. It will be fine. Let's see how the rice turns out.

My mind began to wander. Chip will be home for lunch soon. I want this meal to be good so he'll enjoy it. Suddenly, Chrisi started crying. I went into the bedroom and changed her diaper. Then I picked her up, sat down in a chair, and tried to rock her back to sleep. Finally, she fell asleep. I lay her on her bed and covered her with a blanket.

The rice!

I ran back to the kitchen and immediately turned off the flame. The rice was burning. I let the pressure from the pot come down naturally and then opened the lid. The smell of burning rice rose into my face. I spooned the top layer of the rice out of the pot and placed it in a serving bowl. I tasted some of it. Burned beyond redemption. For some reason—perhaps to confirm that the meal was a complete disaster—I tasted the miso soup. Ughhh! That is truly horrible, I said to myself. How am I going to eat that?

With that, Chip walked in the front door.

"What is that smell?" he said.

"Seaweed," I said, my tone clearly dejected. "I'll make you something for lunch." I made eggs and bacon. I ate a little of the vegetables and as much rice as I could get down. Silently and sympathetically, Chip watched me eat, his appreciation for his food growing with every bite.

After he had finished eating, Chip went back to work. I cleaned up, sat down at my kitchen table, and called my mother.

"This is going to be harder than I thought, *Mamita*. I need your help," I said. "Can you come over and stay with me for a week or two?"

"Of course," she said. "I'll be over later today."

Then I called Bill and explained what had happened. After he'd finished laughing, he gave me the right proportions to cook. He reminded me to cook on low heat, stir little, and time everything at first.

Saved by My Mother—Again

My mother moved into my house and managed to take two weeks off from work. Ostensibly, she was there to care for Chrisi while I devoted the spurts of energy I had to the macrobiotic cooking. Little did I realize at first how valuable her knowledge of cooking would be.

"I'm going to eat what you eat," she announced to me. "We'll do this together." We began by looking carefully at the recipes in my macrobiotic cookbook. My new respect for how difficult this was going to be made me realize that I would have to follow the recipes if I had any hope of getting the meals to be edible. As we paged through the book, my mother would occasionally make comments about the individual foods.

"Oh, wakame. Yes, we called that *luche* in Chile," she said.

"You know wakame seaweed?" I asked her.

"Oh yes. And this one, too." She pointed to the drawing of kombu on the page. "We called this one *cochayuyo*. We used to go into the ocean and harvest both of them. We had many different recipes for these foods."

"Mom, that's great," I said. "Did they taste good?"

"Oh, yes. But we added meat to the dishes," she laughed.

We continued to page through the book.

"*Mote,*" she said. "Barley. Barley is very popular in Chile. It is cooling for the summer. We used to serve it with peaches."

As I listened to my mother's words and her memories of Chile, I realized that she was my link to this new life. She was raised on whole grains, vegetables, beans, and sea vegetables. Yes, in Chile people eat a lot of meat and chicken, but they also eat many plant foods, as well. My mother grew up on these foods and knew them intimately. And now she had come full circle, through me. Macrobiotics had brought her back to her roots. I was reminded of what Michio Kushi had written in *The Book of Macrobiotics:* All traditional cultures were founded on whole grains and vegetables.

"Let's cut up this seaweed," my mother suggested. "We don't have to cook the whole package."

"Let's combine this grain with that bean," she would suggest. "Why don't we boil these vegetables together." At other times, she would say, "These vegetables are very nice blanched." She never failed to come up with good ideas for preparing the food.

And even more, my mother made the cooking exciting and even fun. We laughed at every meal. Whenever a dish was prepared, each of us would look at the other and say, "Why don't you try that one?"

"No," the other one would say, "why don't you try it first?"

And so it went, my mother and me having fun in the kitchen, playing with the food that I hoped would save my life.

In general, the food was bland, at least in comparison to my old fare. We stuck to the basics and avoided even the permitted sauces and condiments. I was afraid to deviate from anything but the purest food, or at least my perception of it. I was also afraid that if we tried something a little bit complicated, we'd mess it up. I wanted to learn how to prepare this food first before I became daring. Chip decided to eat lunch out every day, but to have dinner with us.

As far as the food's possible impact on my health, I did not know what to expect. I hoped it would change my health, but frankly I did not know how it might do that, or what I might actually experience. But one morning, after my mother and I had been eating the food for about a week, I awoke with a surprise: I had no headache. It was gone—gone for the first time in years! In fact, I couldn't remember the last time I didn't have a dull headache. At first I wasn't sure if I was dreaming, or playing some kind of game with myself. I sat on the edge of my bed, as was my custom when I awoke, and turned my attention fully on my head. It was true; I had no headache. That in itself was cause for celebration. One of the many torments that I had had to live with every day was suddenly gone.

A few days later, I awoke, placed my feet on the floor, and clearly perceived that my ankles were stronger and no longer as swollen as they had been. My knees, which had always been weak and swollen, were stronger and largely free of edema. I felt as if I had lost a pound or two, as well. A few days after that, the sores that were regularly appearing in my mouth began to recede. My energy was improving, too.

Was this possible? I had been on the diet for only a week and my health was clearly improving. After ten days, I knew I was getting better. I could not believe what I was experiencing. And yet, there was no doubt in my mind: My life was being turned around!

My mother, on the other hand, appeared to be struck down by a cold or the flu. She had been on the diet for only four or five days when she began suffering from a runny nose, watery eyes, and sneezing. She coughed up a lot of mucous from her lungs, as well. I called Bill and told him that I was getting better, but my mother was sick.

"Don't worry," Bill said. "It's just an elimination of toxins. Your mother is cleansing her system of a lot of old poisons that have accumulated in her liver and lungs. It will pass quickly."

"Is there anything I can do for her?"

"Give her the kuzu tea that you are drinking," Bill said.

"Do you think Chrisi will get it?" I asked him.

"Probably not. Just feed her good-quality food." In fact, I was feeding Chrisi the same foods I was eating, less the salt. I guess because she had very little experience with anything else, Chrisi loved the macrobiotic foods. I would mash them up into baby food for her. She soon developed a taste for tofu, vegetables, and grains and clearly enjoyed these foods.

When I told my mother what Bill had said, she said, "Okay. I'll drink the tea and see what happens." The cold or flu or elimination—whatever it was—passed a few days later. One day my mother showed up at my house after the cold had passed and told me that she felt great—lighter and more energetic. Meanwhile, my sister, who was living with my mother at the time, had adopted the macrobiotic diet and was also experiencing health changes, including a loss of excess weight and a significant increase in energy.

During the next couple of weeks in January, I lost more weight and felt better than I had in years. I was on some kind of roll and I was eager to see Dr. Smith, with whom I had an appointment at the end of the month. We were to discuss the new drugs and the surgery. I couldn't wait to tell him about macrobiotics.

Not What I Expected

I entered Dr. Smith's office for my scheduled appointment filled with excitement. He was sitting behind his large desk, focusing on my paperwork. He looked up, greeted me, and asked me to have a seat. Once I was seated, he began asking me the routine questions that he always did before he gave me a physical exam.

"How have you been feeling?" he asked.

"Very good," I said. "I really do feel much better."

"Oh? Well, that's great," he said. "Have you experienced any changes in your condition since we last saw each other?"

"Well, that's what I want to talk to you about. I want to postpone the chemotherapy and the surgery," I said.

"Why?" he asked me, the alarm rising in his voice.

"Because I have started a macrobiotic diet and I want to give it some more time to see if it can make me well. I've already experienced some small signs that it's helping me."

"You can't do that," he shot back. He got up from behind his desk and started toward me with palpable deliberation. "That food is going to be too hard on you. You're going to hurt yourself. There's not one bit of scientific proof that a macrobiotic diet can do any good."

"How is it going to hurt me?" I asked.

"As your doctor, I can't allow it. You are in a very delicate condition and that crazy diet can only do you harm."

"I have already been doing it and it's helping me some. I want to give it more time," I said.

"You cannot be on that macrobiotic diet. It's crazy and dangerous. I will not go on treating you if you do."

The impact of his words hit me like a tornado. I had been suffering since childhood. Nothing medicine offered me held out the slightest hope for a cure, much less a significant reduction in my symptoms. I had no hope of recovery. On the contrary, if we went ahead with the surgery, I would eventually lose most of my intestines and have an ileostomy bag hanging from my abdomen. What great thing was my doctor offering that permitted him to take such a righteous position? I wondered. I burst out in tears and yelled at him. "This is my only hope," I said. "I need you to support me. This diet makes sense. The food is going into my intestines. That's where the problem is. Look at me. If I make it to thirty years old, I'm not going to have my intestines. This is my last chance and I need you there to help me."

He was fairly shocked by my reaction and backed off. "Okay," he said. "Okay. But you've got to see me more if you're going to go on this diet. And you've got to stay on your medications."

"I will," I said, trying to recover my composure. We agreed that I would meet with him every two weeks and that I would call him if there were any changes in my health.

I left Dr. Smith's office shaken but resolved and even more committed to macrobiotics. No one was going to take away my only chance at recovery. If necessary, I would leave Dr. Smith's care. I did not want to do that because we had formed a bond and he was the only doctor with whom I felt comfortable. But if it came down to a choice between medical treatment, which offered me more drugs and a bag at my side, and macrobiotics, I would choose macrobiotics, the one thing that gave me hope for a new life.

As I drove home that day, I considered Dr. Smith's reaction. Why was it so adamant? I asked myself. What could be so terrible about what I was doing? I couldn't answer those questions for him. But I resolved that if I continued to improve, I would try to help him better understand the macrobiotic approach. Maybe, if it helped me, Dr. Smith could use this diet to help others.

A Test of Faith

Introducing Macrobiotic Cooking became my Bible. I studied that book day and night. I wanted to learn as much as I could about preparing the food and making it as medicinal, if not tasty, as I could. Meanwhile, I started to sleep more deeply and more restfully. I didn't get up as many times during the night, either. One morning, after a particularly good night's sleep, I noticed even more clearly that the swelling throughout my body was being reduced. "I'm on the right track," I told myself. "I am definitely getting better."

The small improvements that I was experiencing served only to strengthen my dedication and commitment to macrobiotics. I had been on the macrobiotic diet only a few weeks and already it was helping me.

And then it all seemed to fall apart early one morning.

One night, late in January, I slept restlessly and was awakened around 2 A.M. by a strong urge to go to the bathroom. There I suffered an acute bout of bloody diarrhea. The diarrhea continued. As it did, I got weaker and weaker. Chip didn't know what to do. He kept on telling me that I had to go to the hospital.

"Call my mother," I said. By the time my mother arrived, I was as white as bleached flour.

"Don't take me to the hospital unless I pass out," I ordered them.

I telephoned Bill Spear but was told that he was out of the country and couldn't be reached. I was bleeding a lot and growing increasingly afraid that I would have to go to the hospital. There must be something I can do to stop the bleeding, I kept saying. Finally, at 3 A.M., I announced, "I'm going to call this Michio Kushi guy in Boston. After all, they're his recommendations that I'm trying to follow."

A woman answered the phone and said in a gentle voice and thick Japanese accent that she was Aveline Kushi, Michio's wife. I apologized profusely for calling at such an ungodly hour, but I was in terrible trouble.

"Oh, it's okay," Aveline said with great sincerity. "We were up anyway." I could hear the sleep in her voice. I thanked her for taking my call and then explained what was happening to me. Fortunately, Bill Spear had already told the Kushis about me and Aveline remembered who I was.

"Let me ask Michio," Aveline said. After a few minutes, she was back on the phone.

"Make very strong miso soup, with extra wakame, and drink a bowl of that every hour until the bleeding stops," she told me. "Then have ume-sho-kuzu." Ume-sho-kuzu was the kuzu drink made with the pickled plum and shoyu.

That's it? I asked myself. That can't be it. Surely you can do better than that. I want the secret formula. I was bitterly disappointed. Not for a second did I believe that food could stop the bleeding. But what else could I do? It was either try the recommendations of the Kushis or go to the hospital. I knew what I would experience at the hospital. It would take weeks to recover from the flare-up and medical treatment.

"Are you going to be around later in case I need you?" I asked Aveline.

"Yes," she said. "We'll be here."

"Okay," I said. "I'll call later, if I need you. Goodbye." I reluctantly hung up the phone.

My mother made the soup and kuzu drink. I did as instructed, drinking the strong miso soup with the extra wakame every hour. By the time I drank the third bowl of soup, the bleeding had stopped. I then drank the ume-sho-kuzu drink and the diarrhea stopped. It was the first time I had ever controlled a Crohn's attack myself and avoided going to the hospital.

Drained and weakened, I was nonetheless relieved and elated. "Oh God, thank you," I said.

From that moment on, I knew macrobiotics was my answer.

6

An Encounter with the Remarkable Mr. Kushi

Chip and I sat in a big conference room in a hotel in downtown Atlanta awaiting the entrance of Michio Kushi, the man who, by all accounts, was the world's leading teacher of macrobiotics. There were about 40 or 50 other people in the audience. They were of all ages, it seemed. Some were hippies, to be sure, but most were professional-looking people, many of them dressed in business suits. Several were clearly ill, but the majority looked healthy to me.

Chip and I sat on the left side of the room, four or five rows from the front. We had driven four hours from Nashville to Atlanta to hear Mr. Kushi speak. This was my first trip away from Chrisi, and even though she was staying with my mom and sister, I was feeling anxious over being away from her. Ever since we left, I'd called my mother regularly, but Chrisi was doing fine, she said. She and my sister were eager to hear what Mr. Kushi was like and what he would say.

Chip and I enjoyed the drive to Atlanta. Chip seemed to open up every time we took road trips and this one was no different. We always grew a little closer when we traveled.

To say that I was excited to be in Atlanta is an understatement. I was desperate for more information about macrobiotics. My mother was no longer cooking with me and I needed to learn how to make the food both tasty and medicinal. Aveline Kushi was scheduled to give a cooking class after Michio spoke and I was eager to attend. As much as anything else, I needed encouragement. Could I do this? I kept asking myself. I now believed that it absolutely would work for me—*if* I could learn to prepare the foods and stick to the diet.

As we waited for the program to begin, I thought about the image I had of Mr. Kushi. I had never met him, of course. In my mind's eye, he was the man who had stood in the shadows behind his wife, Aveline, at three in the morning and told her what I should eat to stop my bleeding and diarrhea. Despite my doubts, his recommendations had worked—miraculously. I marveled that someone could turn food into such powerful medicine. But even more, with that single experience he made me a believer and a follower of his message. Now I wanted to meet the man who had changed my life. He must be tall, I told myself, even though I knew he was of Japanese ancestry and that the Japanese are relatively short in physical stature. He must also have a deep voice and radiate a lot of confidence and power. What will he say? I asked myself. What's going to happen today?

One of the organizers of the event went to the front of the room and introduced himself. He then directed our attention to several people who also were standing at the front of the room. Each of these people had experienced a miraculous recovery through the use of macrobiotics. The first person to speak was a young woman who said she had had a baseball-size tumor in her uterus and was told by her doctors that she would need a hysterectomy to survive her cancer. Instead, she adopted macrobiotics, which caused the tumor to shrink until it disappeared. Her medical tests now showed that she was completely free of malignancy. Not only was she well, but she was capable of having children. Other people with equally remarkable stories spoke about their experiences with macrobiotics. Chip and I looked at each other with our mouths open. "Are these people staged?" I asked him.

An Awakening

Finally Mr. Kushi strode into the room and began to speak in a very thick Japanese accent. He was shorter than I had expected and I had to strain to understand his heavy accent. One of the most distinguishing features about his face was his high and broad forehead. His voice was deep and strong.

"We all come from one infinity," he was saying. "Heaven's force, in the form of cosmic rays and solar energy, comes down upon us in the form of a centripetal spiral of energy." He drew a counterclockwise spiral on the blackboard that began at the periphery and whirled toward the center. "This centripetal spiral is yang," he said. "It causes things to contract or become stressed.

"Earth's force radiates upward." With that, he turned his right hand as if he were spinning a ball between his fingers. "As the earth rotates on its axis, it sends energy away from the earth. That energy moves upward and forms a centrifugal spiral." Now he drew a clockwise spiral that began at the center and radiated outward to the periphery. "A centrifugal spiral makes energy move outward. It causes expansion or relaxation. This is a yin."

"These two forces, yin and yang, flow into the human body—heaven's force from above, earth's force from below." He then drew a man and a woman standing upon the earth. He drew spirals that entered the top of their heads and another set that entered the bottom of their feet. He then showed how the forces of heaven and earth collide within the body and form new spirals where the organs are located. This energy, he said, animates the human organs. Heaven's and earth's forces by their contracting and expanding energy are the life force, bringing life energy and health to every organ, system, and cell.

Earth's force is stronger in women, he said. He reinforced the spiral that entered the woman's body from below. This powerful force causes women to have internal reproductive organs and more developed breasts. Heaven's force, on the other hand, is stronger in men, causing, among other things, external reproductive organs. He showed how the interaction of heaven's and earth's forces caused energy to flow to the eyes, nose, mouth, arms, hands, fingers, legs, and feet.

The human body is sustained by the electromagnetic energy that flows from heaven and earth, he said. It flows through the body in natural and orderly patterns, which acupuncturists refer to as meridians or pathways of energy. Not only does this energy animate every cell and organ, but it maintains our health. As long as it flows unimpeded and abundantly throughout the body, we enjoy radiant good health.

Illness is caused when this energy becomes blocked and imbalanced. When that happens, it becomes excessive in some places and deficient in others. Excessive yang energy causes organs to become overactive, hot, and tired. Deficient yin energy causes organs to become underactive, cool, and stagnant. Such conditions are the basis for weak organ function, accumulation of toxins, degeneration of cells, and eventually serious illness.

Health is achieved by creating balance between heaven's and earth's forces, or between yin and yang. The nature of yin and yang is that they are opposites that continually seek each other and, together, constantly strive to create balance. In a balanced condition, electromagnetic energy flows abundantly throughout our bodies. The universe, Mr. Kushi said, is continually striving to create health, harmony, and balance in everything and everyone. Health, he said, is the natural birthright of humans—as long as we respect and act in harmony with the forces of yin and yang.

Food is the key to maintaining balance between yin and yang, he said. Food is energy, Mr. Kushi asserted. Plants contain solar energy, cosmic rays, and rain water—all manifestations of heaven's force, he said—as well as soil, minerals, vitamins, protein, and fiber, all the products of earth's force. Plant foods, such as whole cereal grains, vegetables, beans, sea vegetables, and fruit are direct manifestations of heaven's and earth's forces. Each food has its own particular balance of yin and yang.

He then drew a long horizontal line on the blackboard. At the left end of the line, he drew a small pyramid, or triangle, with its base at the bottom and called it yang. At the other end, he drew an inverted pyramid, or triangle with its base at the top and its point at the bottom. He called it yin. At the midpoint of the horizontal long line, he drew a small vertical line. This is where balance lies, he said. Whole grains are slightly yang so he placed them on the yang side of the vertical line. Beans are slightly yin. He wrote the word "beans" on the yin side of the vertical line. Root vegetables are a little more yin. Round vegetables slightly yinner, and leafy vegetables yinner still. Fruit is more yin than vegetables. Fruit juice is more yin than fruit. Processed sugar is far more yin than fruit juice; he drew it a considerable distance from the center. He wrote the words for each of these foods on the line to indicate its distance from the center, or from balance.

Fish is more yang than grain, he said. Thus, he wrote the word "fish" a little farther from the vertical center line. Chicken is more yang than fish, eggs are more yang than chicken, red meat is more yang than eggs. Salt is the most yang food constituent, he said. He wrote "salt" at the far end of the yang side of the line.

To maintain health, he said, humans must eat foods that create balance between yin and yang. The best and easiest way to do that is by eating the foods that are more or less in the center of the yin-yang spectrum. That diet is composed of whole grains, a wide variety of fresh vegetables—including roots, round vegetables, and leafy greens—beans, sea vegetables, fish, and fruit. These are the foods that harmonize yin and yang, and thus create balance and health.

The condition of balance, he said, creates the smooth flow of heaven's and earth's forces throughout the body. In this way, electromagnetic energy, or life force, flows abundantly throughout the body. When the life force flows evenly and smoothly throughout the body, all the organs function optimally and health becomes vibrant and strong. Health is the foundation of our lives, Mr. Kushi said. Not only does this electromagnetic energy create health, but it also increases wisdom and spiritual understanding. We begin to better understand the ways of heaven and earth.

On the other hand, when the energy is blocked within the body, symptoms begin to emerge and illness arises. Energy becomes blocked when we take into our bodies extremes of yin and yang. The way most people do this is by eating imbalanced foods and by following an extremely imbalanced diet.

"Strong yang foods, such as meat and eggs, cause contraction here," he said and pointed to the lower organs of the drawing of the man on the blackboard. "Intestines become blocked," he said. "Blood flow becomes poor here and here." Again he pointed to the lower organs and then to the heart. The more we eat eggs, meat, hard cheeses—all yang foods, he said—the more contraction occurs in these organs. This causes blood, lymph, and electromagnetic energy to become blocked and stagnant in these organs, leading to symptoms and then to serious illness. Also, as energy is concentrated in the lower parts of the body, it becomes deficient in the upper parts. "Excess here, weakness there," he said, pointing first to the lower part of the body and then to the upper part.

"Yin foods, such as sugar, ice cream, milk, and yogurt, cause expansion," he said. "They cause energy to move upward and to the outer part of the body—to the skin, central nervous system, and brain. The more we eat these foods, the more energy goes upward and outward—that is yin. As energy goes upward and outward, it becomes deficient in the center of the body and lower organs. That means that sugar and ice cream cause intestines and sex organs to become weak. Soon people cannot assimilate nutrition and digest food. Reproductive organs become weak. Sperm counts fall. Women become infertile. Men and women cannot have children then. Must rely on technology more and more to have children. Humanity is getting weaker.

"If we continue to eat meat, dairy foods, eggs, chicken, sugar, and processed foods, we will get weaker and weaker. More and more people will get sick. Cancer rates will go up even higher. Heart disease, diabetes, osteoporosis, arthritis—all going up. Then medical care getting more and more expensive. More of the country's resources must be dedicated to taking care of the sick. As sickness goes up, judgment gets weaker. We become more and more confused. This leads to more mental illness, social problems, even war.

"Why so many problems?" he asked. "Because we no longer live in harmony with the Order of the Universe. How can we restore our health? We must return to the Order of the Universe by eating whole cereal grains, fresh vegetables, beans, sea vegetables, fish, miso soup, and some fruit. Only in this way can we make ourselves healthy again. As our health gets stronger, we develop greater judgment and deeper understanding of ourselves and each other. This is the way to world peace."

As Mr. Kushi spoke, I started to understand more and more deeply the macrobiotic ideology. And then all of a sudden, the strangest thing happened to me: I had some kind of epiphany. I understood God in a whole new light. I saw why women lose babies, why people become sick, why children are born with disabilities, why violence occurs. I realized that suffering is a consequence of disharmony and that we are responsible for creating harmony, first within ourselves and then within society. God allows suffering as a consequence of not living within the order that He has designed for humans. God isn't remote or inaccessible. He doesn't use suffering to punish us. He provides us with an orderly way to live that promotes health, well-being, and ever-increasing insight into His nature. It is up to us to find that way and live within it. We are free to choose how we live. Somehow, I had stumbled upon that path, which was why I was getting well.

Hearing Michio Kushi speak was like having a door suddenly flung open in my mind and a new understanding flood into my consciousness. I had always felt so much guilt over my illness. I thought that I suffered from Crohn's disease because I had sinned in some way, but I could never figure out what I had done, or why I was ill. Listening to Michio Kushi changed my entire understanding of God and spiritual life. This wasn't about sin and punishment, but about living outside of the natural way that God has created for us. But just as we can live outside of that way and experience the consequences of such a life, we can also return to the way and experience the blessings for which we yearn.

Gratitude and love for "the Creator" overwhelmed me and I started to cry uncontrollably. I was sitting next to the windows, with Chip to my right. I turned away from him and hid my face from those around me. With all my might, I tried to control my sobbing, but nothing could hold back the emotion I felt. Tears of joy, gratitude, and sadness washed over me—joy and gratitude because I had found macrobiotics, which opened the way for this spiritual awakening, and sadness because so many hadn't. Why wasn't this understanding shouted from the rooftops? I asked myself. How could I ever keep this to myself? In that moment, I felt taken up by Spirit, even touched by God.

Suddenly I realized that Chip was concerned and embarrassed by my behavior. He turned to me and said, "What's wrong? Not so loud."

"I'm sorry," I whispered. I could not get the words out of my mouth to explain what I was feeling. And then I went back to crying.

Eventually, Mr. Kushi concluded his remarks and one of the organizers stood up and announced that we would take a 20-minute break. I zealously tried to put into words what I had been feeling so that Chip would understand. He looked at me with confusion and uncertainty. What I said clearly shook his view of life. When the break ended and Mr. Kushi returned to the front of the room, I listened to what he had to say with a whole new attitude. I was hungry for every word he uttered. When he'd finished speaking, he took questions. My head swam with thoughts and queries. I raised my hand and said, "You make it sound like the most important thing is food. How do you explain children with autism?"

"The problem is the intestines," Mr. Kushi replied. "The health of the intestines greatly affects brain function. We must treat the intestines if we want to help people with autism." (Many years later, I would note that on autism web sites a growing number of medical professionals would stress the importance of maintaining the health of the intestines in the treatment of this disorder.)

"Are you saying that these children can be cured?"

"Maybe," he said, "but they can be helped and get a lot better."

Better Than I Thought

That afternoon, Aveline Kushi gave her cooking class. Aveline is the kind of person who absolutely refuses to be placed on a pedestal by anyone. She is continually attempting to humble herself, to make jokes about her forgetfulness or her failures in the kitchen. "Did I put the salt in the rice?" she asked her audience. Then she laughed the most beautiful, self-deprecating laugh possible. "Oh, I'm so forgetful because I drank too much beer last night." This lady was so small and so thin that one could easily imagine that two sips of beer might be too much for her body to tolerate. "I'm sorry," she said. "The beer gave me a runny nose. I get too yang and then I want yin," she said, laughing. "I have to be careful because when I drink beer or eat yin foods, I forget everything that I'm doing and my nose runs." She had the whole audience laughing with her. I realized that she was teaching us about yin and yang by mocking her own foibles.

When she was finished cooking, everyone in the class got little plates of food that Aveline had prepared. The food was delicious. So this is what the food is supposed to taste like, I thought. This is wonderful. Aveline, meanwhile, was apologizing for the fact that the rice wasn't just right, that the beans should have been cooked longer and the greens shorter, that the soup didn't have enough miso. "Oh well," she said with a soft smile. "Next time we do it better."

Even though I laughed through most of the cooking class, I learned so much about how to prepare this food. I also saw how delicious it could be.

That night a party featuring macrobiotic food was held at a house in Atlanta. Everyone from the seminar was invited.

"Let's see what it's like," I said to Chip. "We'll eat some food and leave. Okay? It will give us a chance to experience other people's macrobiotic cooking."

"Okay," he said with obvious reluctance.

It was a potluck dinner at a pretty house in a suburb of Atlanta. When we first arrived, I marveled at the variety of dishes that were laid out on tables in the dining room. Most of the dishes had little cards placed before them that gave the name of the food and listed its ingredients. There were plates full of sushi—rolls of brown rice wrapped in nori seaweed, most with colorful vegetables, or pickles, or noodles chopped up at the center of the rice. There was an endless array of bean dishes, salads, and sautéed vegetables that combined to make every color of the rainbow, it seemed. There were bowls of fried rice, cooked with chopped carrots, scallions, and other vegetables, and various rice and bean dishes. Nearby were burritos and tacos that contained black beans and chopped vegetables. Some of the foods I didn't recognize immediately, but had read about in my cookbooks. These included mochi, pounded sweet rice that was cooked to make a soft dumpling; natto, fermented soybeans used as a condiment on rice; and various seaweed dishes, many of which combined seaweed with vegetables, or seeds, or nut butters. On another table stood rows of beers and bottles of sake. On still another were plates that contained various kinds of cookies, cakes, and a Jell-O-like dessert that was called kanten. I was amazed at the variety of foods and the colors. I was also pleased to note that some of the foods, such as tacos and burritos, were familiar to me.

I had been feeling deprived for more than a month now. And to see this feast laid out before me was not only a revelation—this is macrobiotics?!—but downright exciting.

"Look, Chip, this is what we can eat," I said.

I tried a dish that included tofu and some type of sauce. I had never had tofu before, but the sauce and preparation made it very enjoyable. I have got to learn how to cook this food, I thought to myself.

Chip and I filled our plates with food and then met some of the people at the party. People introduced themselves and said where they were from. When they heard that I was from Nashville, many urged me to start my own macrobiotic center and begin teaching this way of life. My first reaction, at least to myself, was, No way. When I get well, I'm going back to hamburgers and milkshakes. Of course, I didn't say that to anyone.

Everyone I told about my illness encouraged me and insisted that the diet would make me well. Many gave me suggestions for how to prepare my meals so that they tasted better and would still be medicinal. People had such faith in macrobiotics, which moved and inspired me.

Still, the people I met also puzzled me. Most of them ate this way not because they were sick, but because they preferred this food to the standard American diet. How was that possible? I wondered. How could people choose this food over good Southern cooking? It was true that the food at this party was a lot more delicious than the very simple dishes I had been eating. It was also true that Aveline Kushi's meal was wonderful. But could this be a satisfying and enjoyable way to eat for a normal, healthy person? I wondered. I looked around the room and saw people eating the food, talking, and enjoying themselves and I knew that this clearly was a way of eating that many people chose to follow—not because they were compelled by illness or threat of death, but because they were attracted to this food and this way of life.

Early that evening we left the party and returned to our hotel. I felt restless and a bit uncomfortable in my stomach. I had eaten a greater variety of foods than I had consumed in over a month and my stomach was mildly upset. I had a small bout of loose stools, but nothing more. I had a consultation scheduled the following morning with Mr. Kushi. I wanted to get a good night's sleep and be well rested for my appointment. I was eager to meet him.

As I drifted off to sleep, I said to Chip, "I hope I can understand everything he says to me."

The next morning, I entered a hotel room where Michio Kushi and a few of his students sat at a table. I reached out and shook his hand.

"Hello, Mr. Kushi," I said.

"Please call me Michio," he said with a smile.

I told him that I was the person with Crohn's disease who called him at three in the morning. He laughed good-naturedly, without any hint that the call had irritated him.

"Everything you suggested to me that night worked," I said. "The miso soup with the extra wakame stopped my bleeding and the ume-sho-kuzu drink stopped my diarrhea. Thank you so much."

"Good, good," he said. "How are you doing?"

I explained how I was feeling and that I seemed to be making progress. After he asked me what I was eating, I outlined my diet. He made some small adjustments in it. As he spoke, one of his students wrote out everything he said so that I would have a record of his recommendations.

"You're going to be fine," he assured me.

"Do you think I can eventually get off the prednisone?" I asked.

"Yes, yes," he said, "you don't need it." Now he turned to my husband and asked if he had any questions. "No," Chip said.

Very gently, and without any pretension, he told Chip that he had an irregular heartbeat and that his kidneys were overworked. That was the reason he had allergies, Michio said. He encouraged Chip to eat with me. He teased that when we crave something sweet, just give each other a kiss instead.

With that, the consultation was over. Chip and I left the room and as we headed out of the hotel, Chip said to me, "Did you tell him that I had allergies."

"No, of course not," I said.

"Than how did he know that?" Chip asked.

"I don't know," I said.

I was very excited for having met Michio Kushi, but what really impressed me was that he had only fine tuned the recommendations Bill Spear had given me. That gave me even more faith in Bill.

Later that day, I said to Chip, "You know, I think this is going to work for me. If I can make the kind of food we ate yesterday, maybe we could eat this way long-term." During the whole four-hour drive back to Nashville, we discussed how we could fit macrobiotics into our carefully designed life. His parents, the church, and our friends were all of concern.

I returned to Nashville with renewed motivation. Chip and I had attended our first macrobiotic lecture together. He had heard everything Mr. Kushi had said firsthand. Though he didn't say as much, I believed that Chip must have been inspired by Mr. Kushi's lecture, just as I had been. Now he would understand what I was trying to do on a much more personal level. We would be a team now. Our purpose would be to overcome Crohn's disease and enjoy the rest of our lives together. He would have a whole new level of commitment to my healing, I now believed. Not only did he know what I had been suffering, but now he had a much deeper understanding of macrobiotics. Surely he would see how macrobiotics would make both of our lives better. The belief that Chip was now my ally made me feel even closer to him and grateful for his presence. This made me feel all the more that our commitment to each other had deepened, that macrobiotics had become our joint path and not just my own lonely journey.

Crohn's disease is such a lonely illness. It isolates you from other people, because it forces you to become preoccupied with yourself—or more accurately, your intestines—and prevents you from participating in so many social events. You can't go anywhere without taking into consideration the current condition of your bowels. And even when you do participate socially, you have to know just where the bathroom is, in case you suddenly lose control of your bowels or suffer a minor flare-up. Anything can trigger such an event, it seems, even the stress or excitement of being with other people. I remember so many occasions when I was enjoying myself so much that I temporarily forgot my affliction, only to have it arise with a vengeance when I least expected it. One humiliating episode happened while I was driving home from Nashville to Centerville. It was an hour drive. I had made my weekly trip into Nashville to buy my macrobiotic and whole-food supplies. It was late afternoon and I wanted to get home before Chip arrived from work. Chrisi was asleep in her car seat, and I was desperately trying to ignore the rumbling activity going on in my intestines. All of a sudden the sharp pain began. It was so piercing that I gasped for breath. Tears came to my eyes as I furiously looked around for a gas station, a store, or even a house where I could stop and use the bathroom. Unfortunately, I was at the stretch of road that was "country." All I could do was pull over and crouch at the side of the car, just in time. This is no way to live, I thought to myself. I was determined to make this "macrobiotics" work for me.

The Signs Are Changing

By March there was no doubt in my mind that my health was improving. I was sleeping better, my energy levels were higher, and I had lost weight. I wasn't nearly as swollen as I had been. My headaches, which had disappeared after ten days on the macrobiotic diet, had not returned and my joint pain was gone. Meanwhile, I suffered cramping and diarrhea only occasionally and neither of these symptoms ever escalated to their former levels.

I was scheduled to see Dr. Smith for my regular examination. Just before our appointment, he had me go to the hospital and have a blood panel done. The results were sent to him in time for our appointment.

As I walked into Dr. Smith's office, he got up from his desk, walked over to me, and shook my hand. He was holding my medical records.

"How are you?" he asked me. Clearly, he was impressed with my appearance.

"I'm doing much better," I said.

"Yes, you are," he said. "Your blood tests show a significant improvement." He then informed me that my iron levels, which had always been low due to the continual bleeding, had risen. My sedimentation (SED) rate, which was always abnormally high, had fallen.

"Have you stopped the prednisone?" he asked me.

"No, no," I said.

"So tell me, what have you been doing?"

"I've been practicing the macrobiotic diet, as I told you I would," I said. He asked me what that meant, exactly.

I then proceeded to tell him about the diet. I said that it was based on whole grains, vegetables, beans, and sea vegetables. I explained the importance of miso soup and kuzu for the intestines. "The miso has been replacing the intestinal flora that I've lost over the years," I explained. "The flora improves digestion and assimilation of nutrition. Also, both the miso and the kuzu have been promoting the healing of the ulcers and sores in my intestines. I'm not having the diarrhea and the cramping I was before." I then related my experience in January when the bleeding had started again and how I had managed to stop it with the use of miso, wakame, and ume-sho-kuzu drink. I said the diet was having an incredible impact on my health.

"What is kuzu?" he asked me. I explained that it was the root of the kudzu plant, which grows commonly throughout the South.

"So you think the food is doing this for you?" he asked.

"Yes, I know it is," I said.

"The fiber and bulk of these foods are not bothering you?" he asked me.

"I have to adjust the cooking and the quantity of the food," I said. "I also have to use a food mill to limit the amount of fiber in the food. But I have not felt this good since I was a child."

"Okay," he said, "keep it up. Something is working for you, obviously. You look much better and your tests are showing improvement. What can I say?"

I was so excited by Dr. Smith's openness to me that I immediately hurried home, got several macrobiotic books, brought them back to his office, and handed them to him personally. I had visions of him reading the books and using this approach as a way of treating his patients with Crohn's disease and other inflammatory bowel disorders. There was no telling how many people he could help with macrobiotics, people like me who had been suffering most of their lives and were completely at a loss for answers. When I handed him the books, he accepted them graciously. I felt a bond with him at that moment, as if we were discovering something really important together.

As it turned out, it was all for *nada*. A month later, at my next checkup, he gave me back the books. His manner, which had been so open to me before, was now closed shut. His whole personality had changed. He could barely look me in the eye, much less ask me a question about what I was doing.

"Why aren't you jumping at this?" I asked.

"Your case is complex," he replied. "Anyway, I am glad this is working for you. Good luck." With that, he wrote me off. I was devastated.

How could he react like that? I wondered. How could a doctor who treats illnesses for which there are no cures turn his back on a program that was clearly working for one of his patients? How could he keep such information from his other patients who are suffering, especially when all he had to offer were drugs that had terrible side effects and surgery that would eventually eliminate most or all of the intestinal tract?

He continued to see me regularly as his patient, but from that day on, he referred to me as his "miracle lady." He gave absolutely no credence to the diet, nor did he want to know anything about what I was doing. There was none of the rapport that we had previously enjoyed, nor the curiosity that he had initially exhibited about my improvement. When he saw me, he was all business.

At our meeting in March, I asked if I could reduce the prednisone with the intention of eventually going off the drug. He did reduce the amount I was taking, but he was adamant that I remain on the drug. He insisted that the drug was doing me good.

At that point, I had lost so much feeling for him and for the medical establishment that I began to make plans to take myself off the prednisone. In late March, I called Bill and said that I wanted to go off the prednisone and the other drugs I was taking.

"Okay," he said. "But you're going to have to do it slowly and carefully. And it's not going to be easy."

"That's all right," I said. "I'm ready."

7

A Spring Like No Other

The spring of 1980 brought its annual promise of new life, but unlike so many springs before, this one did bear the gift of rebirth. With each passing week, I felt better in body, mind, and soul. I felt as if I was emerging from a long period of darkness and finally coming into the light. In my case, the light had very tangible qualities, not the least of which was the absence of pain.

For a person with Crohn's disease, especially one who has suffered from the illness for many years, pain is a constant presence—not just the acute pain that comes from the abdominal cramping, nor the searing pain that emanates from the wounds in the digestive tract, nor the joint pain that limits your movements. There is also the subtle pain that is a combination of acidic queasiness, intestinal distress, and a deep sense of weakness in your vital center. You are aware that something is eating away at your intestines. Something corrosive, acidic, and relentless is acting on your viscera. And you can't stop it. It's there all the time. You may get some relief through work—during those rare times when you have the energy—or from behaviors that distract you for a while. But the moment you return to yourself and feel your own center of being, there it is again, eating away at you. Every time you sit down to a meal, or drink a cup of tea, or merely relax by a window in the sun, the pain and discomfort resume their hold on your mind. They are all you can focus on. Crohn's disease never lets you forget its presence. It steals your life.

But in the spring of 1980, for the first time since I was a little child, I was being freed from pain. For the first time since I was ten or eleven years old, I was having normal bowel movements. I could relax and allow myself to be aware of my body, without suddenly being aware of pain or the fear of a flare-up. My gut felt balanced and well. I knew I was healing. All of which meant that I was being given back my life. And for the first time since I was a child, I was free to be myself.

But if I wasn't ill, then who was I? I had been sick for so long that I didn't know who I was, or who I could be, without Crohn's disease. Suddenly, I was waking up in the morning with energy and enthusiasm for the day. That was an altogether new experience for me. It forced me to consider what I might do with the day, other than suffer through it, and more important, what I might do with my life. Don't get me wrong, I was ready to experience health. And I was ready to discover who I could be.

That spring was more beautiful than any spring that I could remember. The flowers seemed brighter, the sun stronger and friendlier, the trees more alive and bursting with buds. There were smells in the air that I had never noticed before, colors in the flowers I had not seen in the past, a certain sense of energy in the air that I had not inhaled before. Everything I did that spring seemed far more pleasurable and inspiring than it did before. I even enjoyed my every-day housework, which for the first time I did free of pain. Now imbued with all this energy, I redecorated my house and even put up new wallpaper. I ran errands, took long walks with my daughter, participated in every church event to which I was attracted. For the first time, I allowed myself to believe that I would live a long life and, more important, that I would see my daughter grow up.

The single most consistent emotion that I experienced—if it is an emotion at all—was gratitude. I was grateful, of course, for my newfound health. I was also grateful for being in Centerville. The little town with its beautiful landscapes and rolling hills was just the right place for me to heal, I realized. The pace of life was slow, the people familiar and friendly. There were none of the garish temptations that exist on every corner in the city, such as McDonald's and Burger King, the places I had frequented on a regular basis. Nor were there the sense of alienation and the fear that are so common in cities. Now that I had to stay away from greasy food, I became an observer of the quaint Ma and Pa family diners in "the square" of town. The atmosphere of home and family friendliness was second only to the greasy fried food they served. People seemed to come out of the woodwork to enjoy not only the food, but also the camaraderie. Outside the greasy spoon, it was just as social. Older farmers would be playing checkers, their spittoons set up by their sides. I felt safe in Centerville, and cared about. Yes, this was the place for me to regain my health, I told myself.

The caring that I felt most directly came from my original family—most notably from my father, mother, grandmother, sister, and brother. My whole family adopted the macrobiotic diet as a way of loving and supporting me. They did it, as well, to show how much they believed in what I was doing. My sister called regularly to ask me for recipes and instructions for making a soup or some macrobiotic staple. Every week, my mother popped over to my house with a serving bowl full of soup or rice, or to help me prepare a meal. My father called a couple of times a week to encourage me and to remind me of how much progress I had made. He also began organizing lectures for Bill Spear among his clients and social contacts. In a very short time, my father became so identified with macrobiotics in his community that people were calling him regularly for advice.

My family's encouragement helped me deal with the times when I was discouraged or bored with the food, especially in February and March, before I became adept at cooking macrobiotic foods. In those early months, I wondered if I could actually stick to the diet. At that time, all the food was still very moist and bland. Sometimes it was difficult to keep from cheating, or simply skipping a meal or two. My father knew this and would call me to keep me on the straight and narrow. One morning, for example, he called to ask me if I was eating my miso soup.

"No, Papi, I'm not. I just had a bowl of rice and some vegetables. I'm sick of miso soup," I said.

"Have you made miso soup?" he asked me.

"Yes, I made it. I'll drink some later."

"Why don't you get a bowl of miso soup and have it with me now," he said gently.

"I'm sick of miso soup," I said. "I don't know if I can keep doing this."

"Come on," he said. "Go get your soup. I'm drinking mine. Let's have miso soup together." His words trailed upward, as if he were saying that he was being good and that I should be good, too. "It's delicious. And good for you, too."

"Oh, Papi, don't ask me to do that now," I moaned.

"You know, Ginny, you're doing so well. You're getting better. Let's have some soup together as we talk," he said.

"Oh, all right," I relented. "I'll get some soup."

My family focused its love on my healing—no one more so than my grandmother.

My grandmother was the matriarch of our family. She was loving, and wise, and powerful—and all those qualities existed in her gentle, unassuming manner. She was the most nurturing person I have ever met. Whenever I knew that my grandmother was coming to Tennessee to visit, I would neglect my plants, just so my grandmother could come into my house and say, "Oh, my little granddaughter, look at these plants. Here, let me take care of them." She would water and care for them and in a day or so they would all be full of life again. Then she would go into my flower-bed and attend to my garden, planting new flowers and caring for the existing plants and bushes. She brought the house to life—and me with it. I looked forward to her annual month-long visit, and this time was no different.

As soon as she arrived, she wanted to start cooking for me. Of course, she did not have any training in macrobiotic food preparation. Instead, she used her native intuition and traditional cooking skills. She took care not to use anything but macrobiotic ingredients. "You tell me the foods I can use and I will cook them for you," she would declare. She used her own recipes, which of course came from her own head and heart.

Still, despite all her love for me, I worried about how her meals would affect my health. They were delicious, but were they balanced? I wondered. Concerned, I telephoned Bill Spear and told him what my grandmother was doing.

"Is she using only good-quality macrobiotic ingredients?" Bill asked me.

"Oh yes," I said. "She uses only the foods that I should be eating. But I'm concerned that she might be getting the proportions wrong. Maybe she's using too much miso or tamari, or too much salt or too little salt. Maybe she doesn't cook with enough water. Who knows? My grandmother never had a cooking class and I've only had one."

"Don't worry," Bill said. "As long as she is using the right ingredients and you are getting miso soup, brown rice, and vegetables every day, her food will be fine for you. She wants to help you become well. That intention and all her love go into the food. It will heal you."

Bill was articulating a basic belief in macrobiotics, that family support and love are themselves powerful forms of energy that the human body imbibes, as it were. That loving energy goes into the food, it becomes a part of it, so that when one eats the food, one also takes in the love and intentions of those who prepared the food for you. Rationally, I had no way of making sense of this. All I knew was that the love of my family affected me deeply. It changed my inner state. Whenever my mother or grandmother was cooking with me, or cooking for me, or whenever one of my family members would call, I felt safe and secure, as if I were being held in the arms of angels.

Chip was supportive, in an understated way. He knew very well that my health had improved dramatically on the macrobiotic diet; he was glad I was feeling better; but he never spoke much about the changes the diet had caused in my life, nor in his own. Those changes were significant. For years, he had been taking biweekly injections to treat his allergies, but after a few months on the macrobiotic diet, the allergies went away and he stopped the injections. His energy levels increased, he lost weight, and the heart palpitations that he had suffered periodically went away. Yet, all of these changes seemed to make only the most superficial impression on him, a fact that baffled me deeply.

Chip found the macrobiotic philosophy interesting, in a passing sort of way, but he had little interest in applying that philosophy to daily living. The cooking and the enormous body of knowledge that connected food to health held no fascination for him at all. The contrast between the two of us could not have been greater. I was utterly captivated by the macrobiotic understanding, which of course has its roots in Asian philosophy and Chinese medicine. The body of knowledge that formed the foundation for macrobiotics was thousands of years old. It could fill many libraries and I wanted to know it all. For me, this knowledge was developed by people who were interested in the most essential things in life: health and illness, longevity, the purpose of life, and the relationship between spirit and matter. An important link in the macrobiotic lifestyle is the preparation of food. There is a natural order to how food affects our bodies. Cooking is necessary to release food's properties. Through cooking, you bring these factors together in a balance that affects your quality of health. By taking ownership of your food choices and the way you combine and prepare your food, you create energy and balance for your body. This became evident to me when I would eat out. My choices of food would be healthier, but the energy of the cooking, the restaurant environment, and the cooking method caused me to feel less energized than when I ate my own cooking at home.

Somehow, Chip didn't see things in the same way I did. Consequently, we talked about his work, our schedules, church activities, and daily events more than we did about my health. He continued to eat my cooking, and when he felt that he needed "real food," I made him the kinds of foods he liked or he went out.

As for my husband's parents, they were detached from me and what I was doing. Form and manners were very important to my parents-in-law. They reacted to things as if from a distance. For them, it was good that I was feeling better. As long as my macrobiotic diet didn't hurt their son, or get in the way of their relationship with their granddaughter, it wasn't a problem. As it turned out, all of that would come later.

The progress I made that spring convinced me that the time had come for me to take the leap that I was terrified of, but desperate to make. I wanted to go off the prednisone.

Shaking Myself Free of the Crutch

Bill came down to Tennessee that April ostensibly to give lectures on macrobiotics. The real reason for his visit, as far as I was concerned, was to help me develop a plan to free myself from the drugs. In addition to the prednisone, I was also taking Azulfidine and potassium. (I had already given up the diuretics when my weight dropped and I stopped taking the aspirin when my headaches disappeared.) The Azulfidine and potassium were milder by far than the prednisone. I planned to go off them after I had weaned myself off the prednisone.

Bill was very careful about the prednisone. I had been taking the drug for five years at that point. My system had adapted to it. He knew that I would have withdrawal symptoms. If I didn't take precautionary measures, he said, those symptoms could be severe.

From the macrobiotic point of view, all drugs have both short- and long-term side effects. Some are experienced while taking the drug. In the case of prednisone, those short-term side effects include headaches, joint pain, enormous fluctuations in energy levels, puffy cheeks, swelling, glazed eyes, and weight gain. But there are also long-term side effects, which include damage to the liver and other organs. Of greater concern for the moment, at least according to Bill, was that residues of the drug had been retained in my system. As I weaned myself from the prednisone, those residues would start to be purged, or "discharged," from my tissues and released into my bloodstream, where they would trigger symptoms. These discharges would become even more severe when I gave up the drug entirely. Bill cautioned me that if I didn't reduce the doses of the drug slowly and carefully—and thus allow my system to gradually purge the drug—I could suffer a rapid and violent discharge that might bring about severe symptoms, the likes of which he could only guess. Only later in my healing process would I understand the full impact of his warning.

Bill and I made a meal plan that would help me get off the prednisone. He wanted me to eat kuzu with my meals to strengthen my intestines. He taught me how to make kuzu with squash and kuzu with vegetables. He also recommended that I drink ume-sho-kuzu three times a day to keep my blood alkalized. I was also to eat seaweed, especially nori, which he said would stabilize my nervous system and reduce some of the symptoms. Both the kuzu and the seaweed would keep my blood alkaline, which would promote the strength of my immune system and balance the prednisone. He also wanted me to eat very well, to drink whenever I was thirsty, and to maintain healthy bowel elimination, which was how I would eliminate the drug residues.

Just before I attempted to give up the drug, I underwent a series of blood tests and met with Dr. Smith. Much to my happiness, all of my blood tests were normal, including my SED rate. During my session with Dr. Smith, I told him of my plan to get off prednisone. As before, he was adamantly opposed to such a step. "Why don't you get to a low level and stay on the drug for the rest of your life?" he asked me.

"I want to know for sure what's making me well," I said. "How much of my improvement is the drug and how much is macrobiotics? I know this diet is making me better. I want to know if I need the drug at all now. Maybe I don't. And if I don't, I want to live drug-free if I can."

In early May, I began the job of reducing my daily doses of prednisone with the intention of eliminating the drug completely. At first, I lowered the dosage by reducing the number of pills I took each day, but pretty soon I had to physically cut the pills into pieces to get the right amounts.

The big hurdle was 10 mg. I had read that at 10 mg, the symptoms of withdrawal become more intense. I also worried that as the doses got lower, the Crohn's disease might return. Surely, that's exactly what would happen if the disease was being controlled by the prednisone, I admitted. But how would I discern the difference between withdrawal and the return of the Crohn's disease? I wondered. How should I interpret diarrhea or a flare-up? I kept asking myself. Will it mean that I am suffering withdrawal symptoms from the drug or that I still need the drug to control my illness? Needless to say, I was both confused and afraid.

At that point, I did what I always do when I'm afraid: I prayed. I asked God for help and strength and to see me through this difficult time. Meanwhile, I kept cutting up the little white pills, holding each pill with a tweezer and slicing off smaller and smaller pieces with a knife. As the pieces became smaller, I used a magnifying glass to determine if they were the right size and dosage.

It wasn't easy. I felt like a mad scientist, hovering over my tiny pills with my knife, tweezers, and magnifying glass, hoping to get just the right dosage in my weaning process. After I got below the 10 mg threshold, I became extremely careful of how small the dosage could be. Ten milligrams was too high now; five was too low. I kept shaving the pills until I got below 5 mg and then I stopped them entirely. That's when the symptoms began to emerge. And when they did, they hit me with a vengeance.

One of the first problems to arise was loose stools, which immediately triggered my fear of a flare-up. The nausea returned, as did the stomach cramps. My mouth became very dry. I sucked on ice cubes to quench my thirst. As all of these symptoms arose, I was sure a flare-up was on the way, but my symptoms never escalated to that level of intensity. Still, the pain had just begun. For three days, I suffered periodic bouts of the jitters in my hands, arms, and legs. Then my headaches returned, but this time they were different and very odd. I could feel heat and a sensation that I can only describe as pressure coming up my spine. The pressure would spread into my shoulders and then fill my head with pain. It felt as if my head had been placed in a vise that someone was tightening. The pain gathered behind my forehead, eyes, and cheekbones. It felt as if it would never leave, but after a couple of hours it would start to ease. The headache would be followed by a deep cold that would settle into my bones and cause my entire body to shake. I would shiver for short periods—20 to 30 minutes—and then the symptoms would fade, only to return a few hours later. Afterward, the old restlessness would return. I developed insomnia again and spent much of the night sweating profusely. I got hot flashes and then cold sweats. I felt as if I had been plunged into menopause. At night, I would move onto the couch to avoid keeping Chip awake. I would bury myself under blankets when I was cold and throw them off when I was hot. In between, I would read a book and wonder how long all of this would go on.

In the midst of these symptoms, my emotions seemed to go out of control. At intervals, I was angry, frustrated, and weepy. I yelled, cried, and paced the room as if I were a caged animal. Desperate, I sometimes got into the car and just drove around Centerville, hoping to distract myself from my emotional turmoil.

All of this occurred during a single week, but after four or five days, the symptoms were clearly subsiding. I had stopped the prednisone on a Monday and by Friday I experienced a clear reduction in the severity of all the side effects. By Sunday night, they were gone. I thought that once the withdrawal symptoms had passed, I would be filled with energy and feelings of good health, but nothing like that happened. That weekend, I became very quiet and introverted, as if I were protecting a wound that was healing. I felt well, but tender and sensitive. My mood became mellow and soft. I felt a tremendous sense of relief. A fog had lifted, it seemed. By Sunday afternoon, everything seemed right with the world. I didn't have to do anything but simply live and enjoy the balance in which the world rested.

About a week later, I gave up the Asulfadine, which did not

cause the same intense withdrawal symptoms that the prednisone had. By the end of May, I was drug-free. My Crohn's symptoms did not return.

Reborn

That summer, I began a new life. For the first time since I was
nineteen years old, I was not taking any drugs. Moreover, I was
free of all my symptoms of Crohn's disease, as well as of Takayasu
arteritis, though the latter disorder had represented more of an
abstract fear than a day-to-day impediment to my life. Once I was
free of the drugs, my life seemed to open up. I had ambitions
and dreams again. Late that spring, I even thought about going
back to school in September. Why not? I told myself. I'm healthy.
Indeed, I had more energy and vitality than I had had since I was
a child. All of the residual puffiness, bloating, and weight that
had clung to my body as a result of the prednisone had left me
when I gave up the drug. That summer I even wore a two-piece
bathing suit and looked good in it. That was no small accom-
plishment for a woman who stood only five feet two inches and—
just a few months before—had weighed more than 140 pounds.

Once I was off the drug and my Crohn's symptoms were gone,
my libido returned, as well. That was no small miracle. First, it
improved my marriage tremendously. Chip was not an attentive
person, which meant that sex was one of the primary ways we experienced closeness and affection. As I said, for a woman with
Crohn's, the libido is virtually nonexistent. But even worse, sex itself can be very painful. Chip and I regularly fought about sex,
especially when I was not feeling well and he desired sex. Don't
get me wrong, it was not his fault that we had sexual problems.
He was healthy and naturally wanted to make love to his wife. But
I was ill and sex could be painful and difficult for me at times, especially when my symptoms had been flaring and any pressure
against my reproductive organs was painful. The truth was, Chip
and I were in very different places when it came to sex and neither one of us could be blamed. But once I was off the drugs and

my body was healing, my sex drive returned. Also, I was physically healthy, which meant that sex was no longer painful. Sex brought us closer and gave us greater physical and emotional intimacy. Even if Chip didn't say very much, he and I both longed for the closeness that sex gave us. A barrier that had existed between us for years was melting away. It was that spring of 1980 that I began to think about having another child.

The change in my libido did more than just improve our marriage, though. It changed my perception of who I was. I don't mean to be abstract about this, but I discovered that my sexual libido restored my sexuality, which I experienced as a kind of energy that influenced my entire being and gave me a stronger sense of self. It was as if I had a greater sense of personal power. I found that as my sexual energy rose, my identity became stronger. I felt fuller, more alive. These feelings had little to do with sexual arousal, in fact. Rather, they had more to do with the return of my sexual identity, and thus were a part of my everyday life. For the past six years, my sexuality had been lost as a consequence of the disease. That meant that something vital and alive had gone out of my life. Now that my vitality and aliveness had returned, they seemed to infuse my every cell. They added to my experience of health. Being healthy, I realized, was being whole.

One way of understanding wholeness is to see it as a kind of integration between all our parts, so that everything from our spiritual life to our sexual identity exists in a state of acceptance and love. Because all our disparate parts live in such a state of harmony, they are influenced by each other. Nothing is rejected, and yet everything finds its correct place and its own correct sense of proportion in our lives. As my health improved, I felt more whole, more integrated, and more grounded on the earth. As my energy levels rose, I felt more relaxed and at peace with myself.

Of course, my entire church community recognized the transformation I had undergone. Most of the people at my church were very supportive of my diet and lifestyle, though most thought of it as a terrible fate that had to be suffered. "Oh, you poor thing," many said. "You have to eat that."

"Oh, it's not so bad," I told them. "I've actually learned to enjoy the food. Besides, it's making me well," I would say.

My recovery was not lost on the other people who were suffering from illness. By late spring, people were coming to me regularly for advice on treating their health problems. Looking back, I realize that it was that summer of 1980 when I started teaching. It started informally, of course. People would just start asking me questions about this or that disorder from which they suffered. I had no medical background at all, but I very much wanted to help people. The only thing I could think to do was to read as much as possible about macrobiotics and its approach to various kinds of illnesses and then explain what I knew. It wasn't much, but it was something I could offer.

That summer, a local dentist who had long been a promoter of organic foods and a more natural lifestyle told us that his daughter had been diagnosed with breast cancer. She had been sick for some time but was now interested in starting macrobiotics to help herself heal. The church community rallied around her and several macrobiotic potlucks were held to support her in her recovery. She had surgery and chemotherapy, but the macrobiotic diet diminished the side effects of the drugs and boosted her energy levels considerably. Her parents were very grateful for my help, as was the community. The woman's illness brought our community together, and for the first time, I felt a bond with Centerville. I also felt a tremendous responsibility to learn all I could about macrobiotics.

All of this had an odd effect on my relationship with my husband. Chip didn't want to be seen by our community as someone who had to eat a macrobiotic diet. Nor did he want to be restricted by it when we were in social situations. He wanted to eat what everyone else ate, and to be seen as someone who ate like everyone else. That was fine with me. The problem was that he wanted me to eat like everyone else, too. When we attended a social gathering and there were no foods available that I could eat, Chip would become upset and tell me privately, "Don't just not eat. Try something." On the occasions when I brought my own foods, he felt self-conscious and uncomfortable. "Do you have to take your food this time?" he would ask me. "Can't you just eat what everyone else is eating?"

Chip was more supportive of me when we were alone, but when it came to social gatherings, he wanted us to be a "normal" couple, which in his mind meant eating "normal" foods.

Of course, his perspective left me scratching my head. "Don't you remember what I've been through these last five years? What *we've* been through?" I would ask him. "I can't eat those foods. I get sick. Remember?"

Somehow, in Chip's mind, my diet was fine at home, but inconvenient outside the home. He didn't understand that I couldn't flip a switch and be able to eat barbecue at a picnic and not suffer the consequences.

Of course, this revealed how little Chip understood the role of macrobiotics in my life, as well as the extent of my suffering with Crohn's disease. Even though he had been with me through all of my pain and frequent hospitalizations, those experiences didn't seem to sink in very deeply. He didn't comprehend the depth of my illness, nor how much it had affected my life. There was no way that I was going to risk going back to those days. As for macrobiotics, Chip saw the diet as just another form of medicine. Once I became well, I should be able to eat anything, he believed. In that regard, I couldn't blame him. Through the first few months of macrobiotics, I maintained the same perspective—namely, that as soon as I got my health back, I would resume my old way of eating. But as I remained on the diet and experienced its healing powers, I began to realize ever more deeply that there was no going back. I would only become sick again. I also realized that if I allowed myself to become deeply ill again, I might not be able to get back my health a second time. Health was life itself to me now and macrobiotics was the source of my health.

With Spirit Beneath My Wings

That summer I attended a week-long macrobiotic summer camp in the Pocono Mountains in Pennsylvania. My mother went with me to help care for Chrisi while I attended classes. My cousin Sylvia also came from Connecticut to attend. My family was impressed with how well I was improving on the macrobiotic diet and they were individually starting to show interest.

At the camp, I took my first really intensive cooking classes and for the first time began to understand and appreciate the art of macrobiotic cooking. I marveled at the diversity of the macrobiotic foods and how much could be done to make them flavorful, delicious, and satisfying. This was a cuisine that was intended to be delicious. It was not a deprivation diet, as I had long believed, but a way of living that could be just as rewarding and satisfying as the typical American diet. The big difference, of course, was that the macrobiotic foods were intended to satisfy the palate while also giving health to the body.

There were many things that I was exposed to at the macrobiotic summer camp that took time to understand or accept. The macrobiotic philosophy of yin and yang was still largely inscrutable to me. I knew that this part of the practice would take time and study, so I let it be.

The basic underpinning of macrobiotics was Oriental philosophy, which emphasized balance. Michio Kushi maintained that every religion, including Judaism and Christianity, taught the use of food as a way of maintaining health and fostering spiritual development. Indeed, he even pointed to many interesting stories and quotes from both the Old and New Testaments that strongly supported his views. As one who reads the Bible regularly, I was impressed not only by the soundness of his thesis, but also by his insight into the Bible.

As I had learned when I was in Atlanta, people who followed the macrobiotic diet came from all strata of society. Many were using the diet to heal themselves of illness, but many had come to it simply because it supported their health and appealed to their psychological and spiritual natures. No matter what their motivations for adopting the diet were, however, most people whom I met eventually came to a new understanding of themselves and a greater spiritual awareness as a result of their macrobiotic practice. For the most part, people who followed macrobiotics placed enormous value on spiritual development, which they saw as more important than accruing material things. They saw the dietary practice and the cultivation of health as essentially spiritual practices. Good health gives rise to good judgment and a sensitivity to the higher human values and aspirations, macrobiotic people maintained. The more one ate whole grains and vegetables, the more sensitive one became to the subtle, finer vibrations that make up the universe. Meat, cheese, and sugar, on the other hand, burden the body, especially the nervous system, making us increasingly insensitive to the subtle energies that are present in all of life, including those gentle and oftentimes hidden feelings inside of us. As people become more out of touch with their inner and outer worlds, they become increasingly materialistic, at least according to what macrobiotic people believed.

All these ideas caused me to reflect on my own beliefs and values. I began to see myself as a far more materialistic person than I had previously realized. Like so many other people in my little church community, I saw myself as very caught up with the pursuit of middle-class values and the acquisition of material things—nice houses, cars, and clothes. The contrast between my values and those of many of the macrobiotic people whom I met at the Pocono summer camp revealed how arrogant I was. In the past, I did not see how spiritual life might influence the foods I choose to eat or how I choose to dress. Indeed, before macrobiotics, my diet and clothes were influenced to a great extent by social trends and pressures, rather than by how I felt deep inside. The macrobiotic philosophy maintains that everything we do, especially the foods we eat, influences our spiritual development. Could eating this simple food give me a stronger feeling of connection to God? I wondered. Maybe it could. I did feel my values changing since I began eating this way. And that summer I felt a strong need to grow spiritually. I wanted to open up to new possibilities and to become simpler in my way of living. It was a kind of epiphany for me to realize that simple living could make me more sensitive to the finer rhythms of nature and better able to listen to the gentle voice inside me. I believed that God was answering my prayers by presenting me with macrobiotics.

All of this strengthened my sense of spiritual connection to God. During my youth, my grandmother was my spiritual teacher and the one I turned to for spiritual guidance. After I got married, I turned to my husband for that guidance, but he was very reluctant to be the spiritual leader of our family. I wanted him to lead the family in prayer and to provide me and our children with spiritual direction. "Just because we don't pray together doesn't mean I don't pray," he would say. He was right, of course. Macrobiotics taught me that every person must develop his or her own private relationship with God. I could not turn to others, not even to my husband, for something that could be felt or experienced only within me.

Going Beyond My Reach

By the middle of August, I reached a peak in my health. I was brimming with energy and confidence. It was then that I decided to register for four courses in the Special Education Department at the George Peabody School at Vanderbilt University in Nashville. I was determined to resume my education, to pick up my life at the point where it had been diverted by disease. I had two more semesters to complete to get my degree. Once I was finished with college, I could be a teacher of disabled and handicapped children. That had been my ambition before I became sick. Now that I was well, I was more ambitious than ever.

My course load required that I be at Vanderbilt three days a week—Monday, Wednesday, and Friday—starting at 9 A.M., for an early morning class, and finishing at around 5 P.M., for my last afternoon class. The George Peabody School is an hour and a half from Centerville, which meant that I would have a three-hour commute each day. Chrisi and I would drive in to Nashville each morning, where my aunt would take care of her while I was in classes. My mother would help with Chrisi after she returned home from work. Still, that was a long day, I realized. But I was well and Chrisi would be fine, I told myself. And I was finally resuming my life.

Little did I realize that there was still a lot I had to learn about health and balance.

8

Learning the Hard Way

The minute I set foot on the George Peabody campus on August 14, I felt as if I had stepped into another life. I strolled among the great halls of learning and joined the hustle of other students hurrying to class. I rubbed shoulders with professors and broke into my new books with both trepidation and excitement. I had great energy and enthusiasm for learning and for life. I was proud of myself, because I had made it all the way back. This is where I had left off five years before. Now I was resuming my studies and my life was back on track. Once again, I was among ambitious people who were working hard to fulfill their dreams. I was one of those people now. But I was more, too, because I had so much experience now and had overcome so much adversity. At the same time, I felt young and ready to take on new challenges. Those first couple of weeks at George Peabody were one big adrenaline rush.

It was during that time that I saw Dr. Smith for another one of our regularly scheduled visits. He examined me and noted that my latest battery of blood tests—including my SED rate—were all normal. As far as he could tell, I was in good health. But as we concluded our appointment, he looked at me in a strange way and said, "Be careful. This may not last."

On the one hand, that was a cruel statement, especially to one who had suffered for so long. But on the other hand, it was prophetic. Of course, at the time I was oblivious to such nuances. I shrugged his comment off and left with a smile on my face, pretending that it was just concern that he was expressing. I was on some kind of high and the thought of things turning downward never even occurred to me.

Inevitably, school and my schedule became more demanding. It seemed as if I was running from morning till night. I had to be in the car by 7:30 A.M. so that I could be at school by 9:00. If it was Monday, Wednesday, or Friday, I had to attend classes throughout the day; on Tuesdays and Thursdays, I had my practicum. Once I got home at night, I had to cook dinner, take care of Chrisi, and do my homework. When Chrisi was in bed and my homework was finished, I prepared breakfast and lunch for the following day. This schedule had to be maintained day in and day out, the only letup being on the weekends.

In the middle of September, Chrisi got sick, which meant that I had to stay home for a couple of days. That only created a backlog of work, which put even more pressure on me. It wasn't long before I was falling behind and the first thing to start slipping was my diet. I found myself eating in vegetarian restaurants or trying to make the best choices in typical American places.

By about the second or third week in September, I felt my energy levels fall. I had greater difficulty getting out of bed. I was tired during the day and wanted to go to bed early at night. At first, I fought the awareness that my body was flagging. I pressed on, thinking that it would be only another couple of months and the semester would be over. If I kept pushing, I told myself, I would find the stamina I needed and eventually the fatigue will pass. But it didn't. By the end of September, nothing that I was doing was fun anymore. I had several papers that I had to turn in to my professors and tests were starting. Meanwhile, I had become increasingly uncomfortable deep inside myself. One day I got out of bed in the morning and realized that I was losing weight. Thanks to the macrobiotic diet and getting myself off prednisone, I had lost all of the excess weight that I had carried for the past five years. My weight had finally stabilized and fluctuated only slightly, ranging from 105 to 110 pounds, which was where I was comfortable. But one day in late September, I realized that my clothes were loose on me and then it hit me: I'm losing weight. But why?

At that point, I should have known that I was in serious trouble and that I had to turn back to a simpler, more health-promoting lifestyle—and fast. I needed rest and good food. I needed to stop pushing myself and neglecting all the signs that I was acutely out of balance. I had been too active and too stressed. All of this had created an elevation in my stress hormones and too much contraction in my muscles and organs. In short, I was too yang. I needed to make balance with my lifestyle by slowing down, getting more rest and relaxation, and letting go of the tension that had gripped my life. I should have paid greater attention to my physical and psychological needs, among the most important of which was to spend more time with my family, especially my daughter. All of these influences, of course, were yin, which in the macrobiotic philosophy would make balance with my extremely yang lifestyle.

None of that happened because I didn't let it happen. Instead, I just pushed myself harder. And each day, it felt like I was walking against greater and greater resistance.

The effects on my body started to snowball. By early October, I began to have loose stools, which soon turned to diarrhea. Frantic, I called Bill Spear for advice on how to stop the diarrhea. He recommended a couple of medicinal drinks. I did not tell him of my schedule, however. I was afraid that if I mentioned it, he would insist that I leave school, which I was not prepared to do.

By the end of October, I had a full-blown flare-up, with uncontrollable diarrhea and a low-grade fever. Both the diarrhea and fever were extremely debilitating. They drained me of energy. I felt like a limp dish towel. By Halloween, I could not get out of bed. Much to my horror, my weight had fallen to the mid-80s. I made more calls to Bill who gave me more recommendations. I did everything as instructed, but the diarrhea continued sporadically and the fever persisted.

Soon, I developed a strange set of bumps on my legs. Bill thought that they might have been caused by my not assimilating my food and nutrition properly.

I knew that I could not continue in school so I got a leave of absence. My teachers sent work home to me. Initially, I intended to keep pace with my courses, but that was just a fantasy. I soon realized that I was simply too weak to do any of my schoolwork and had to withdraw.

The thought of going to Dr. Smith hovered in the air, but I refused to do that because I knew what it meant. He would order me to the hospital, where I would be placed on IVs and prednisone.

On some level, I was denying what was happening to me. I kept asking Bill if this was a discharge, meaning that my health was actually improving, that my body was eliminating old toxins. Bill was equivocal. He clearly didn't like the signs, especially the fact that the fever was not going away. He gave me a number of odd remedies, including a tea that had among its ingredients a small clump of hair from my husband's head. Nothing worked. By the first week of November, my weight had fallen to 78 pounds and I was clearly ill.

Finally, Bill called and suggested that I come to Connecticut and stay with him and his wife, Joan, for a short while. If I was directly under Bill's care, I could get the right foods, medicinal teas, and other forms of support that offered the best chance of healing. Bill explained that I could stay at his house for a week and then at a nearby study house, where he provided housing for some of his students.

At that point, I realized that I had to do something. Either I went to Bill's house or I went to the hospital. I chose to go to Bill.

Chip, Chrisi, and I flew to Connecticut, where we met my father and Aunt Virginia at my father's house. My father drove us to Bill's house in Middletown. Once there, my family and I all stood outside of Bill's house and said our goodbyes. One by one, I hugged and kissed my loved ones. And then suddenly it hit me: I was sick and about to be alone to try to heal myself. I didn't want to be alone now. I wanted my mother and grandmother.

Instead, I was going to be with Bill and his wife, Joan. They would not love me like my family. I didn't know what they would expect of me, but in the end, I would have to make myself well. It was all on me. I didn't know if I could make myself well again. I grabbed Chip and started crying uncontrollably. "I don't want to go," I said. "Don't make me go. Let's go back. I'll go to the hospital." Chip consoled me and reminded me that this was where I wanted to be.

As soon as he said that, something inside of me realized that I did not want to go to the hospital, even though I didn't want to go to Bill's house, either. Gradually, I regained my composure and understood that this was inevitable. My Aunt Virginia took Chrisi into her arms. Virginia lived just outside of Stamford and would keep Chrisi for the next two weeks. My family seemed to line up a little distance from me, as if collectively letting me go. I turned toward the door to Bill's house and everyone waved goodbye. Bill let me into the house and the door closed behind me.

The Long, Dark Tunnel

I entered Bill's house through the kitchen door and immediately saw that the kitchen was long and narrow, with counter tops on either side and pots and pans hanging from a rack above. I met Joan Spear. She was just a little taller than me, perhaps five feet four, with dark eyes and hair. Joan and Bill escorted me through the house, which was very clean and neat. The living room contained simple furniture and a lot of exposed wood. A long table with perhaps ten chairs occupied the center of the dining room. Bill showed me to my room. It was spare. My bed was a futon that lay on the wood floor. A chair sat in one corner. A small chest of drawers stood against one wall. He left me to unpack. When the door closed, I sat on the chair and felt completely and utterly alone.

I realized that Bill and Joan were taking on a tremendous amount of risk and responsibility when they took me in. I was sick, feverish, and emaciated. I had terrible diarrhea that could have escalated into even more severe symptoms. Any normal American in my condition would be in the hospital getting IVs and drugs. Bill knew the risks involved and he was very cautious with me. Before I came to Connecticut, he explained that he was going to do everything he could to help me recover, but that I would have to comply with everything he told me to do. This was not going to be easy, he had said, and it wasn't going to be particularly comfortable for me, either. I would have to rebuild my health and strength. That was no small challenge in my condition. Only the strictest diet and life-supporting behaviors could give me back my health.

Soon I heard a knock on the door. I opened it and Joan walked into the room. We made some polite conversation and then she said, "You know, why don't you give me your makeup and perfume. You shouldn't wear any of those things here."

"You can't take away my makeup," I said.

"It's no good for you," she said. "Those chemicals are going into your skin."

"At least give me my mascara," I said. The thought of going without my mascara shocked me. All my cultural inclinations about a woman's appearance suddenly surfaced. A Spanish woman doesn't go without making up her eyes, I thought.

"There's no one to impress here," she retorted.

I grabbed my mascara and handed her the rest of my makeup. She took them and left.

A little while later, I came down for dinner. About five other people from the macrobiotic community had come over to eat with Bill and Joannie. Eventually, everyone gathered in the dining room and took their seats. Just before I took mine, Bill pulled me aside and told me that he would rather I didn't speak during the meal. I should concentrate on chewing my food thoroughly so that every mouthful was turned into a liquid before it was swallowed. "Some of the people will be around after dinner and you can talk then," he said.

"All right," I said. But this was another blow that upset me. I took my seat with everyone else and thought that being here was becoming increasingly harsh. Everyone was now passing serving bowls and plates around the table. Bill and Joan had put aside a separate set of bowls for me. My food was simpler than that of the others at the table. There were no sauces for me and fewer condiments.

My meal was composed of brown rice, two forms of green vegetables, a root vegetable, seaweed, and miso soup. Though the vegetables and seaweeds would change each night, the basics would remain essentially the same. That first night, I tried a condiment that Bill referred to as natto. It was made of fermented soybeans that had a very sticky, stringy glaze over them. Whenever you picked up the natto with your fork or chopsticks—the people at Bill's preferred to eat with chopsticks— long strings of the glaze remained attached to the condiment that was still in the bowl. You had to swirl the natto in the air to get the strings to let go of the remaining condiment in the bowl. I placed some on my rice, as the others were doing, and tasted it. Ughh! Horrible. It had a strong, pungent flavor that I found revolting. I looked around and saw that everyone else was eating it with alacrity. There was no doubt that they were enjoying the food immensely. How could they eat that stuff? I wondered.

I ate in silence as everyone else talked in an unrestrained way. A young man who was seated across from me turned and asked me what my name was.

"This is Ginny," Bill said. "She's going to be staying with us for a little while, but she's not talking during dinner. She needs to concentrate on chewing her food thoroughly. You can talk to her, but please don't ask her questions during the meal." I smiled weakly and the young man smiled back.

I suddenly felt extremely self-conscious and restricted, as if I were mute or somehow handicapped. Meanwhile, I concentrated on chewing my food and turning every mouthful into a liquid. At first, I couldn't chew the food for very long before I swallowed. But as I concentrated on chewing, I found that I could chew more and more until the food was fully liquefied. Eventually, I could chew a single mouthful of food 150 times before I had to swallow it. That became my practice. I found it had a powerful affect on both my experience of the food—the food became sweeter and more delicious the longer I chewed it—and on my body—I felt lighter after the meal and slightly stronger, in fact.

Once the meal was completed, we cleared the table and socialized a bit. I was exhausted and went upstairs to my room. I closed the door behind me, lay down on my bed, curled up into the fetal position, and cried my eyes out.

After the first night, my father came often to have dinner with me. Since I had to chew, he would do the talking, telling me about the cute little things Chrisi had done and said. Hearing about my daughter and how well she was doing reassured me and nourished me, too. I yearned to be with her. As we sat at the table, my father's loving gaze would occasionally meet mine. In that instance, he would communicate so much warmth, compassion, and concern for me. Sometimes I wanted to just get up from the table and hug him forever. His strong, loving presence was my anchor in the storm that was raging inside of me.

Every night, Chip would call and fill me in on the details of what was occurring in Centerville, as well. How I longed to be home with him and Chrisi. I needed him to tell me every little thing that was happening there. I was desperate to be reminded of the life I had left only a few days ago and to which I would soon be returning. One night, Chip called me and told me that Connecticut was where we needed to be. That's where I could get Bill's counseling and Joan's cooking classes. Connecticut was where my health would be restored. This was Chip at his very best. He was telling me that he would pull up stakes and move our family to the place where I would get the best care possible. But Centerville specifically, and Tennessee in general, was our home and the place Chip loved. To force him to sacrifice all that Centerville meant to him would be wrong. Besides, I told him, I felt no special affinity for Connecticut anymore. I would get well while I was here and be all too happy to come home to him and Chrisi.

But Chip's gesture only made me miss him and our home all the more. After getting off the phone with him that night, I experienced another intense wave of memories, emotion, and purging.

I realized later that at Bill's house I let out a lot of emotional pain that had been building up inside me for months, probably even for years. I cried most of the nights I was there. It seemed silly to me at times. Why do I feel the need to cry so much? I kept wondering. I'll be here for only a few days. Soon I'll be reunited with my daughter and Chip. What's the big deal? But then the emotion would rise inside me again and out it would spill in a flood of tears. I didn't hold it back. I just lay there and let it out.

Oddly, each of these episodes was associated with different memories, many of them very difficult. I had been sexually molested during childhood, once in Chile by a farmhand and again in high school by a teacher. I associated these experiences with terrible fear, anger, confusion, shame, and guilt. Now, for reasons that I could not explain, these horrible events and their related emotions forced their way into my consciousness. For years, I had kept them at bay, repressing the images and emotions every time they had tried to surface. Here at Bill's house, I could no longer repress them, perhaps because I was in a weakened state, or because something within me insisted that they be fully restored to my consciousness. The tears I cried now came from deep in the pit of my soul. I wasn't just remembering, it seemed to me, but reexperiencing these events and purging myself of them. It felt as if these events were coming up from the basement of my soul. And as each memory came bursting into my consciousness, I went through convulsions of emotion. Invariably, the fear emerged in all its horror, followed by intense anger and rage. These feelings were followed by overwhelming sadness, which itself would be transformed into compassion—first for myself, but then for people everywhere who have suffered at the hands of more physically powerful figures. As these paroxysms overtook me, my breathing caused my chest to heave and fall, as if I were physically expelling something from my body. Finally, after hours of crying, I arrived at a state of exhaustion and peace. I felt as if I had been at sea during a raging storm and was finally thrown up on a safe shore.

What was causing these powerful emotional outbursts? I wondered. It had to be the separation from Chrisi and Chip, I told myself. But each night, when I went upstairs to my room and tried to sleep, I would be visited by some ghost of the past that would torment me for hours until, exhausted and empty, I finally fell asleep. I experienced many other difficult and conflicting emotions, such as my love and anger for my father, whose infidelities represented a kind of abandonment of my mother, me, my sister, and my brother. Mistakes that I had made came into my memory. I remembered the time Chip and I had run away from home when we were teenagers. Our parents had been pushed to the edges of their sanity looking for us. The guilt I felt for causing them such pain was intense and terrible. Now, being a parent myself, I would begin to understand their desperation. Every night at Bill's house, more waves of emotion overtook me. It was as if I had a movie playing in my head, showing me the events of my past life in detail. The pain of emptiness would then take over and leave a hollow, cold place deep inside me. I also grieved the miscarriage I had when Chrisi was ten months old and my conditions were beginning to flare. It was all part of the illness, I told myself. But the desire for another baby became unquenchable. It wasn't until I had passed through all these emotional states that I was finally released into sleep.

After a few days at Bill's, I began to feel stronger. My diarrhea came under control, but my fever lingered. On the third day I was there, Bill brought me to a medical doctor in Hartford by the name of H. Robert Silverstein, who had an office at St. Francis Medical Center, a large hospital in the center of Hartford. Dr. Silverstein was a cardiologist and an internist who had a general medical practice. He gave me a full examination and ran an array of blood tests on me. In addition to using conventional medicine, he also used diet and herbs to treat people. Dr. Silverstein found that, in addition to my persistent fever, I had an irregular heartbeat, my liver was inflamed, and in general, my organs were stressed. My blood tests, however, were all normal. He prescribed a number of herbs, which he said would break the fever.

After the examination, I thanked Dr. Silverstein and we returned to Bill's house, where I took Dr. Silverstein's herbs. One of the things that Bill insisted on was that I wear only cotton clothing, which he said would help my skin to breathe more freely and promote the circulation of energy throughout my body. That limited my wardrobe some and I ended up wearing only the simplest clothes at Bill's. Also, there was nothing to do during the day. Joan was busy cooking and doing her housework. Sometimes she would iron in her sewing room. There was a television set there and I ended up sitting on the floor and watching television with her at times. There was very little conversation between us.

A couple of days later, I lay in bed at night and started sweating profusely. I literally drenched my clothes and shivered intensely. But in the middle of the night, the fever finally broke and the next morning I felt better than I had felt in a couple of months. There was no doubt about it: Bill and Joan's food, the behaviors that they insisted I follow, and Dr. Silverstein's herbs were working. I was clearly getting better.

On my last night at Bill's house, I was awakened from sleep by a knock on my door. I called out, "Come in." Bill entered the room with a tall, strongly built Japanese man. Bill introduced him to me and told me that he didn't speak much English, but that he was a very gifted Japanese healer. Bill wanted him to do some energy work on me. Would that be all right? he asked.

"I guess," I said. I had no idea what an energy healer was. "What is he going to do?"

"All he's going to do is put his hands on you," Bill said. "You don't have to do anything. Just lie there and be comfortable." Bill nodded to the man and said, "It's okay. It's okay."

The man understood, knelt down beside me, rubbed his hands together and placed his hands on my body, one hand on my solar plexus area, the other on my lower abdomen. I had never experienced anything like this before. I felt self-conscious and a bit tense. The man closed his eyes and seemed to be concentrating very deeply. Suddenly, through my clothing I could feel heat radiating from his hands. It was a very comforting heat that penetrated deeply into my body. I couldn't get over how good it felt. My body started to relax. I felt as if I was drinking in the warmth. Soon I fell off to sleep. I must have slept for only a few minutes because when I awoke, he was still over me, his hands in the same places. As before, I experienced the heat that radiated from his hands and through my clothing. I dozed again; I couldn't help it. When I awoke, he was still there working on me. I wondered if by sleeping I might have prevented the good that he was doing for me, but his concentration never wavered and he remained unchanged through the entire process. I knew that I should not talk or ask him any questions. I decided to pray. My prayer was different. I found myself praying from deep within myself. I felt somehow that a deeper part of my being had been opened. My prayer was filled with gratitude. It wasn't my usual fearful and desperate prayer. I was thankful for everything up to that point in my life. I was thankful for this man and his abilities, for his generous willingness to help me. I was thankful for Bill and Joan, who had taken me into their home to care for me. Soon I was asleep again. The next thing I knew, it was morning. I woke up feeling full of energy and absolutely wonderful. The Japanese healer seemed to fill me up with something—"energy" was the only word I could put to it—that was still with me in the morning.

Into Phase Two

That day, I packed up my clothes and moved into the study house. There I was greeted by two women and two men, all of whom were living at the house and studying macrobiotics with Bill. The house was bigger than Bill's and older. There were about six bedrooms. As soon as I walked into the house, I got a warm, relaxed feeling. It felt good to be here. One of the women, whose name was Mary and who worked at the house as a cook, greeted me with a warm, almost motherly love. Mary was large boned and slightly heavyset, with beautiful skin, bright eyes, and a big smile. I thought that all macrobiotic people were skinny and it was good to be with someone who had a more traditional, heavier build. That night, she began to administer ginger compresses on my intestines.

A ginger compress is made by grating ginger root into a cheesecloth pouch (just a square of cheesecloth that is tied off at the top) and placing the pouch in water that has been boiled and is still very hot. A towel is dipped into the water and allowed to soak up the ginger water. The towel is then twisted from both ends, allowing the excess water to run out, and then placed over the part of the body that is suffering from some disorder. The ginger compress causes an abundance of blood to rush to the area of the body over which it is placed. The blood brings immune cells and nutrients to the organs that are weak or in need of healing. The heat also causes the blood to circulate more rapidly in the area. The blood moves into and away from the area to take away the heat and thus takes away any toxins that may be accumulating in the organ. The ginger increases the warmth and acts as a kind of irritant, causing even more blood to flow to the area.

Receiving a ginger compress is very relaxing and comforting. But Mary's love seemed to come through, as well. Her warmth was mixed with that of the compress. I felt as if I were being attended to by an old friend, someone who cared about me.

During the middle of that week, Aunt Virginia brought Chrisi to me. I had been longing for this visit since I had turned Chrisi over to Virginia. I held her in my arms and never wanted to let her go again. That afternoon, Chrisi and I played and cuddled. Every little thing she did pulled me closer to her. I kept kissing her and telling her I loved her. Very gently, I tried to explain that I was feeling better and that we would go home in just a few days. She didn't react to my words because she was only 20 months old, but she was happy that we were together. But at the end of the day I had to turn her over to Aunt Virginia. Chrisi let out a little whimper and then a small cry, but Virginia, who is very loving, kissed her and reassured her. Once Aunt Virginia's car disappeared down the street, I went into the house, lay on my bed, and fell into another long, lonely cry.

After a while, I went downstairs and encountered John, one of the residents of the house, who asked me how I was doing.

"I just had to let go of my daughter," I said. I burst into tears again. John was so gentle. He took me by the hand and led me into the living room, where we sat down on the couch. He put his arm around me and at that point, I just started talking about how difficult all of this had been—my illness, my practice of macrobiotics, my stupid desire to return to school, my stubbornness when my body tried to tell me to slow down, and my relapse. I told him about being at Bill's house, the loneliness and the progress, and how all I wanted now was to take my child into my arms and go home to my husband. My every word was wet with tears.

John sat there and listened with complete attentiveness and sincerity. He said nothing; he just listened. And when I was finally spent, when my tears had dried up entirely, he gave me a few minutes to recover in silence. Then he took my hand and placed a small sculpture of an owl in my palm.

"What's this?" I said.

"That's an owl," he said. "In native American mythology, the owl is believed to make the sun rise. You hold this owl and your sun will rise again." With that he gave me the owl and a comforting hug.

My eyes welled up again and I said, "Thank you so much." He didn't realize how much hope his words and actions had given me. Since that day, I have loved collecting owls.

By the end of my second week in Connecticut, all of my acute symptoms were gone. There was no fever, no diarrhea, no cramping. I was weak and needed rest, but I could get that at home. Chip flew to Connecticut to pick up Chrisi and me. But before we returned to Tennessee, we reunited with my entire family at my father's house, where we celebrated a big Thanksgiving feast. We had turkey and many vegetables and squash. My grandmother made miso soup that included turkey-broth, vegetables, and seaweed. "I made this special for you, my little granddaughter," my grandmother said. No soup was ever more delicious.

How wonderful it was to be back in the cocoon of love that was my family.

Back Home—To Other Problems

Chip, Chrisi, and I went home to Tennessee. I was so weak, I had to be escorted through the airport in a wheelchair. Bill sent a macrobiotic cook to live with us for two months so that I could rest and recuperate without having to cook my meals. He had given me strict instructions: Rest, sleep, eat well, play with your daughter, play with your husband, and regain your strength. I could do all of that, I had said.

My mother came to my house the morning after we arrived back in Centerville. I was weak and wanted to take a shower, so I asked my mother to help me get into the tub. She helped me get undressed in the bathroom. When I had all my clothes off, she looked at me and started crying.

"What's wrong, Mom?" I said. My mother never cries. She's so strong, yet so caring. It always seemed to me that my mother could hold the entire world—with all of its suffering—in her eyes and still smile and encourage people. And though she tried to hold back the tears, she was unable to.

I turned my head and caught the image of myself in the mirror. Suddenly I, too, was shocked and horrified. I had no shape. I was down to 78 pounds and had lost all semblance of my adult, female body.

"You look like one of those children in the television commercials who are starving," my mother said, crying. "Have you thought about this? Are you sure you are doing the right thing?"

I felt her fear for me. I also felt no small amount of my own.

"I'll go to my doctor," I said to reassure her. "If he wants me to go to the hospital, I will."

"Yes," she said. "I think it's a good idea."

I postponed my trip to Dr. Smith in the hope that the macrobiotic cook would help me recover my health sufficiently that I would not have to see him. I knew that as soon as I saw Dr. Smith, I would wind up in the hospital again.

The macrobiotic cook was an expert, precise in her cooking and very generous with her knowledge. She prepared light, strengthening foods for me and hardier, richer fare for Chip and Chrisi. Her food was delicious and healthful. I was getting stronger by the week, and as I did, I began to help her prepare the meals. And then my in-laws came to stay in our house the week before Christmas. They would be there for the next few weeks. I had spoken to them on the phone and reminded them that we were eating vegetarian. They would need to bring a few groceries for themselves.

The two arrived with bags of groceries in their arms, dumped them on my kitchen counter, and proceeded to unpack steaks, frankfurters, bacon, eggs, ice cream, cheese, and milk. It wasn't long, of course, before they started cooking these things. I had been eating well for nearly a year by then and was extremely sensitive to the smell of food. Suddenly, the smell of burning flesh filled my house. I went into the kitchen and found my mother-in-law cooking sausage. This was no surprise, as this was a typical part of their breakfast. I looked at her. She was impassive, distant, certain of herself. She was making a statement and a stand.

My parents-in-law had always maintained a cool distance from me—they were cool, inexpressive people in general—but they also communicated their severe doubts about my macrobiotic practice. Now that I was ill, they expressed even greater doubt about what I was doing. Perhaps they felt that the diet had created my current health crisis. Still, they knew that it was the diet that had helped me overcome my Crohn's disease. That should have been enough for them to recognize how important it was to me. But it wasn't and now they were implying that it would hurt their son, Chip, and perhaps my daughter, too.

Fine, I told myself. Let them have the run of the house and let them eat what they want. They'll be here for only a few weeks.

That was not the attitude of my macrobiotic cook, however. She found the cooking of steak, sausage, bacon, and the like not only unpleasant, but intolerable. Like me, she detested the smell of flesh cooking. But she also maintained that the grease that was on those foods would remain on my pots and would leach itself into the macrobiotic foods that she and I were eating. She also hated the thought that that same grease was in the air and would be taken into our bodies through our skin and breath. She found the sharing of the kitchen with my mother-in-law unbearable.

The same could not be said for Chip. He ate his mother's food with a passion and, in effect, had returned to her kitchen. She cooked all three daily meals for him and he ate each with abandon. You might think that that bothered me, but it really didn't. I wanted it known to both my parents-in-law that Chip was free to eat as he wished. I was not forcing him to eat macrobiotically.

Chrisi, on the other hand, was a different story. My parents-in-law wanted to give her the same food they were eating themselves, which upset me because my daughter had been raised, for the most part, on whole grains, beans, vegetables, and seaweeds. There was a limit to how much of the high-fat, high-protein foods they could give her without her getting sick. They also wanted to ply her with ice cream and sugary candy. Every child likes ice cream, but Chrisi had not eaten dairy foods and I did not want her to have too much. Also, this was December—cold foods are not appropriate in the winter, my macrobiotic practice had taught me—and she was only 21 months old. Eating a lot of ice cream wasn't good for her. I felt the same about candy and chocolate. My father-in-law didn't like being told that, however. He wanted to give her the foods that he was used to eating and he didn't want me to get in the way.

I knew that I had to give everyone some latitude. Otherwise, we were going to have real trouble in the house. But I didn't want Chrisi to get sick. I had to find some kind of middle ground with my parents-in-law. I asked both of them not to give her ice cream or candy until after she had eaten her usual macrobiotic dinner. I felt that if she ate a good meal first, the sweets wouldn't have the same harmful effects. Nor would they ruin her appetite for good food.

The cook found all of my parents-in-law's behavior intolerable. "You're ill," she kept telling me. "We have to provide good food for you. How can I do that if they're cooking sausage and steak in your pots and pans and filling the house with grease?

That quality is in your air. It's on your pots. You're consuming that food, whether you like it or not," she told me. "I do not want to eat that food. If something isn't done soon, I will have to leave."

It wasn't just the food that my cook found unbearable. It was also the conflict that was gradually escalating in our house. Clearly, my parents-in-law were making a stand against my diet and way of living. In a way, they seemed to be taking back their son and their granddaughter.

I tried as best I could to keep the peace. As often as I thought possible, I tried to explain macrobiotics to them, but they turned a deaf ear to me. Every time I tried to justify my macrobiotic practice, they were like two stone walls. They didn't want to hear it.

The Façade Blows Away

You could cut the tension with a chisel. Finally, the cook had had enough. She could no longer share the kitchen with my mother-in-law, she couldn't stand the smell of burning flesh, and she hated the attitudes of both my parents-in-law toward the food and toward her. One day she woke up, made breakfast, and announced that she would be leaving. She would make enough food for me for a few days, she said. All I had to do was reheat it. Once that was done, she was going home.

That, of course, just increased my own stress. I was weak, tired, and feeling the conflict with my parents-in-law even more now. I had lost my only real macrobiotic ally. Chip had maintained a kind of ostensible neutrality; he didn't want to overtly support me on the diet, or in my silent battle with his parents. Up until the time my parents-in-law had arrived, I thought that Chip and I had an understanding about macrobiotics. I had tried to explain to him just how important the diet was to me and how I thought Chrisi needed the healthy foods, as well. At home, Chip supported me with the food and didn't express any reservations about feeding Chrisi macrobiotic foods. But things were very different when his parents were around. All outward signs of support from him vanished. He could not stand up to his parents, and when they took a stand against the diet and me, he remained outside the fray, which is to say, he silently sided with them. Meanwhile, the atmosphere in my house became more tense and conflicted. It clearly took a toll on me.

I went to see Dr. Smith just before the holiday. He was visibly shocked to see me in such a debilitated condition. He believed that I had an abscess from the Crohn's disease in my intestines and told me that I should go immediately to the hospital. I told him that I would go right after Christmas. When I returned home, I started to make plans to enter the hospital. The first thing I had to do was to make arrangements for my daughter. I knew Chip's parents would want to take care of Chrisi while I was in the hospital. My mother would be able to make the foods I wanted her to eat. In the meantime, I wanted Chip's parents to cut down on the foods they were giving her.

"Do you think it would be okay if I asked your mother if she would not give Chrisi so much snack food?" I asked Chip.

Chip wouldn't answer me directly. He didn't want to ask his parents to cut down on the ice cream, candy, dairy foods, and meat they were giving Chrisi, but he wouldn't say specifically that I couldn't do it, either.

"Okay," I said. "Why don't you send your mother in and I'll talk to her."

Chip's mother came into the room.

"I know that you don't understand what we're doing with food, but this is the food Chrisi has grown up on, and if she gets too much of the food you're eating, she'll get sick. I don't want you to go to too much trouble, but if she gets sick, it will be more trouble."

Chip's mother reacted with cool detachment. She became more distant, even remote.

"Okay," she said, as if she were speaking to the wall. "If this is what you want. But I won't be able to give her the foods you want. I don't know how to prepare them. I won't be able to do it right."

"Just limit the amount of sugar and dairy food you give her, okay?" I said. "That's really all I'm asking."

Suddenly, Chip's father entered the room with a distinct air of combativeness.

"What's going on?" he asked.

"I was just asking Mrs. Harper if she could limit the amount of sugar and dairy food that she and you give to Chrisi," I said. "Chrisi has been raised on macrobiotic food and I'm afraid that if she gets too much of these other foods, she'll get sick; they create too much congestion. I don't know how long I will be in the hospital but I don't want you to have a sick baby on your hands."

His entire body stiffened.

"I am sick and tired of you controlling everything around here," he said. "It's okay if you need this diet for your condition, but you shouldn't be imposing it on everyone else. It's not working for Chip. He's lost weight, for God's sake. And you're going to turn your daughter into a freak. She's going to be different from all her friends in school. If you need medicine for your diarrhea, than you should take it, but stop making the rest of us have to live with it."

"I know you don't understand this," I said and burst into tears. "Chip is not doing this because he has to. He is giving me support. He doesn't have to eat this way. He's choosing to eat this way."

"I shouldn't have to ask your permission to feed my granddaughter something," Chip's father shot back. "If I want to give her ice cream, I should be able to do that. I shouldn't have to ask you first or be on some kind of schedule with it," he said. "You just go on to the hospital and we'll take care of our granddaughter the way we see fit."

Suddenly, I was overcome by desperation. I looked over at Chip for some support, but none came. Mrs. Harper reassured me that she would watch the foods she gave Chrisi and I shouldn't worry.

Feelings of being alone, ganged up on, and fighting for my daughter and my own life overwhelmed me. I was too weak, tired, and ill to fight with them now. All I could do was break down and cry. Once they saw that I had turned away and was unable to go on fighting, they all left the room. I tried to gather my emotions and my wits. I'll do what I have to do for Chrisi, I thought. I'll make sure my mother prepares some of Chrisi's meals.

The Most Important Choice of All

On December 27, I entered the hospital, where I would remain until January 2. I was placed on an IV and made to undergo a full battery of tests to determine, among other things, whether I had an abscess in my intestines. The tests showed that there was no abscess, much to Dr. Smith's surprise. That wasn't all they showed. According to my barium enema and colonoscopy, there was very little inflammation in my intestinal tract now. Clearly, my small intestine had healed a great deal since I began the diet. Virtually all of my blood tests, including my SED rate, were normal, as well. My only negative sign was that I was anemic, which the doctors corrected in the hospital by giving me vitamin B shots and iron supplements. Dr. Smith insisted that I resume the prednisone. I negotiated with him for the lowest dose possible. He agreed to start me out at 10 mg, but with the intention of going back up to 45 mg.

Despite the generally positive news about my intestinal health, I felt no sense of victory. I was overcome by exhaustion and sadness. I kept going over the fight I had had with the Harpers and how Chip had failed to support me when I needed it most. I felt as if the life force had drained from me entirely and that my very existence hung by a thin thread. One night, as I lay in my hospital bed, I felt myself letting go of that thread. It was as if the will to go on living lifted out of my body, like a bird leaving its nest. Without any words forming in my head, I knew in some deep place inside of me that I could let go right now and leave this life behind me. A feeling that gave me permission to die arose inside of me. I felt it clearly. I could say yes to the silky darkness that was calling me forth. My body started to relax. I surrendered and slid toward the abyss. For an instant, there was a pause, a void, a thoughtless emptiness.

No! The word jolted me back into consciousness with the power of an electrical shock. It was as if some bigger force, one that was both inside of me and outside of me, sent an electrical pulse through my being and shifted me back into physical existence. Every fiber of my being, every cell in my body, shouted that word, *No!* This is not my time, this is not the way I am to die. Just as I had known only a moment before that I was letting go of my life, I now knew with even deeper certainty that I was alive and meant to live. This was not how my life was to end, a voice inside me shouted. There is more for me to do. There is more of this life to live.

9

Dawn

I returned home to a temporary peace. Dr. Smith had me increase my prednisone by 5 mg every other day until it plateaued at 45 mg. I accepted that I had to be on the medicine, at least for now. But as before, the side effects arose almost immediately. The two most palpable effects on me were hunger and energy— I had lots of both. No matter what I ate, I was still hungry. After I got out of the hospital, of course, I was very thin, so I did not view the hunger with any immediate alarm. I thought that as long as I was so desperate to restore my weight, I might as well keep eating.

Meanwhile, I also had an abundance of restless energy, as if I had taken ten cups of coffee intravenously. Prednisone creates a kind of anxious energy. Your body feels off-kilter, shaky, and charged with a low-grade fever. All you can think to do with these feelings is to distract yourself with work or other activities. You do anything to keep from feeling the shaky fragility of your body. To a great degree, I could counteract these feelings with my macrobiotic diet, which gave me some relief from the anxiety, but the feelings of restless energy were almost a constant.

About a month after I got out of the hospital, my husband's best friend got married in Florida. The couple invited us to stay with them at their house for a few days before their wedding and we accepted. Once we were in Tallahassee, we were swept up by an endless parade of parties. It seemed that my husband's friend had a multitude of friends and associates who wanted to celebrate as much as possible before the wedding. There were also several rehearsals for the wedding, all of which managed to turn into parties. At every event, there was an abundance of hors d'oeuvres or full-scale meals, all of which triggered my appetite and served as compelling temptation. I resisted as best I could, but it was a battle. Little by little my prednisone-fueled hunger caused me to indulge in this food and that one. I struggled against my hunger, and it seemed that my hunger struggled against my will. The more I ate the food, the more my body seemed to want it. Soon, I was at war with myself, indulging in foods that I knew were no good for me, and suffering small recriminations from my inner voice afterward.

Meanwhile, Chip and I were not getting along very well. He made small, critical comments about me to his friends, even as I stood among them. Very often, these comments were made as jokes, but they stung me, nonetheless. Increasingly, I felt insecure and vulnerable, especially with Chip. I found myself wanting Chip's attention and approval more than usual. I also felt my will to resist all the food that was around me getting weaker and weaker. I didn't have the support of having my macrobiotic food around. It made it extremely difficult to ignore all the food around me.

And then there was an odd and off-putting theme that was occurring in the house where we stayed. The soon-to-be married couple were very public, even loud at times, during their lovemaking. One night, as Chip and I lay in bed, we were treated to a concert of verbal outcries emanating from the bedroom across the hall.

"Why isn't sex like that for us?" Chip said to me as we lay awake. "Why aren't you like that," he said, referring to the woman who was rather outspoken in her pleasure.

"Well, you need to find out what he's doing," I said to him.

Of course, such conversations get two people nowhere, which was where we ended up that night, lying back to back, hopelessly lost for answers. Still, these small insults, as well as my insecurities and raging hunger, were taking a toll on me. The next morning, I woke up as if possessed. Before anyone else got up, I got into the car and drove to a local waffle house, where I ordered two enormous breakfasts that included eggs, bacon, toast, grits, hash browns, waffles, sweet rolls, and hot chocolate.

"Are you expecting someone else?" the waitress asked me.

I then proceeded to eat everything I had ordered. Finally, I experienced some satiation of my out-of-control hunger. A kind of food-induced intoxication settled over me. I ate more as if trying to fill a void. As I did, I could feel the eyes of every waitress and patron in the place looking at me. Their collective judgment hung in the air like the heavy breath of a jury. Meanwhile, I ate. And ate. And ate.

When I was finished, I was lost in a kind of hypnotic state. I felt the sweet greasiness of the food swell within me and push against my skin. I was utterly humiliated by what had happened and could barely look up from the table. I paid the check, got into my car, and cried the entire way back to the house where we were staying.

I wanted desperately to talk to someone about what had happened, so when I got back I told Chip.

"Why did you do that?" he asked me, exasperated. Was he afraid that I was going to get sick and ruin the rest of the time we would be in Tallahassee?

"I don't know," I said. "I couldn't help myself."

Chip had no understanding of this; neither did I. After a short initial exchange, we both retreated into our respective shells and said no more about it.

Later that day, I was overcome by fear of the possible effects the food would have on me. I didn't have to wait long to get my answer. Within 24 hours, the food combined with the prednisone to create a sudden rash of symptoms, the most notable of which was that my stomach swelled to the point that I looked three months pregnant. I went from being thin to being overweight in less than 48 hours. Within the next few days, I noticed that my old chipmunk cheeks popped out again. I also went through

strange, periodic bouts of perspiration. On the other hand, I had
no symptoms of Crohn's disease. No attacks of diarrhea, cramping, or bloody stools occurred. At first, this made little sense to
me, until I remembered the results of my hospital tests: The doctors had found very little inflammation in my intestines, which, I
surmised, must be the reason I had no obvious Crohn's attack
after my binge.

Still, I longed to get home to my miso soup and brown rice.
On the drive back to Nashville after the wedding, I began to
make plans for restoring my health completely and getting off
the prednisone once and for all. There were two things that I
had to do when I got back, I realized. First, I had to eat exceed-
ingly well. Second, I had to stay home with Chrisi and maintain
balance.

The reason I had gotten into so much trouble the previous
fall was clear to me now: I had tried to do too much too soon. I
had exceeded my limits by miles. This caused me enormous
stress and made my condition excessively yang. It was pure arro-
gance. I had lost myself to my unfulfilled ambitions and the lin-
gering frustrations that had arisen after my last college year was
taken from me. But I was no longer nineteen years old. I was a
mother; my child needed me at home. Indeed, I saw my respon-
sibilities in an entirely new light. I realized that the realities of my
life were exactly what I needed to maintain my health and balance, because they described a lifestyle that was conducive to my
health. The inescapable truth was that life had provided me with
what I needed to heal. If I ran from my life to fulfill my old fan-
tasies, I would rob my daughter of a mother and wind up sick
again. It was time to embrace the truth of who I was. I was more
than ready to do that.

Preparing for Another Leap of Faith

After I'd settled in and reestablished my routine of cooking
and eating macrobiotically, my health soon became even stronger
than it had been before the fall of 1980. My body felt balanced

and stable, even in the face of the prednisone. I lost the excess weight that the drug and my Tallahassee binge had caused. My energy levels were consistent and I suffered little anxiety. I had no symptoms of Crohn's. Meanwhile, I continued to study macrobiotics, nutrition, and health. The stronger my health became, the more I wanted to help others who were ill, especially those with Crohn's disease.

That spring of 1981, I invited Bill Spear to Nashville to give lectures on macrobiotics. While in Tennessee, Bill adjusted my diet and told me how good I looked. I was making tremendous progress, he said. Not only was that music to my ears, but in some place deep within me, I knew it to be true.

"I am going to go off the prednisone again, Bill," I told him.

"Okay," he said. "You know what to do."

We went over a plan to support my health while I weaned myself once again from the drug. Once that plan was ready, I went back to Dr. Smith and told him that I was committed to getting off the prednisone. He expressed his usual caution. He gave me the lowest possible dosage, but urged me to stay on the drug indefinitely. In June, I decided to wean myself off the drug. As had happened the first time I got off the prednisone, I suffered an array of familiar symptoms, including a few days of cramping and diarrhea. All the symptoms passed quickly this time.

That spring, all of my blood tests were normal. I had normal digestion and elimination and no symptoms of Crohn's disease. I have never had to take prednisone again, nor have I taken any other pharmaceutical agent for Crohn's disease. I have not had a single attack of Crohn's since 1981. Speaking from my experience and the many tests I have undergone, I am completely free of Crohn's and have been for twenty years.

That summer of 1981, I became pregnant with my second child, much against the advice of my doctors. In March of 1982, I gave birth to a healthy baby boy, Hyde Spain Harper IV, or Buddy as we call him. My pregnancy with Buddy was sheer joy. I kept my weight to the usual pregnancy weight. My appetite was healthy, and with the Crohn's symptoms gone, I was able to enjoy a wide variety of healthy whole foods. I was feeling wonderful and this little life inside me filled me with renewed energy. The pregnancy and delivery went smoothly. Chip and I were old pros now and we enjoyed every phase of the event. Chip was proud to have a son and I was proud to give him one. The doctors had wanted to put me back on the prednisone as a precaution just during the last part of the labor and delivery. I refused, agreeing only to go on the drug in case of emergency. Holding Buddy in my arms brought total fulfillment to my life. His angelic face held so much promise. I kissed him all over as I told him, "You are living proof of my perseverance and hope. You are the bright light at the end of my dark tunnel. You were worth it all!" At the time of this writing, Chrisi is twenty-two and Buddy is nineteen. Both are healthy, normal young adults and continue to follow the macrobiotic principles.

One Last Goodbye

Despite the fact that I no longer suffered from any Crohn's symptoms, I did have to endure another health crisis, courtesy of the prednisone. Two years after I gave up the drug for good, I developed a series of large welts, or skin eruptions, on both my calves and shins. The welts, known as eurothema gangranosis, were discharges of the last remaining residues of the prednisone from my tissues and liver. They were extremely painful. At times, I could hardly walk for the pain.

I went immediately to my doctor, who told me that the welts were extremely dangerous. If they were not controlled, they could eat away enormous patches of skin. I could lose both tissue and bone and, if not dealt with properly, I could even lose my legs. My doctor wanted to put me on a drug called dapsone, which was so toxic that I would have to undergo regular tests to see if it was destroying my liver.

"Let me go home and think about it," I told him.

"Don't fool around with this," he said. "Your macrobiotics is not going to be able to do anything about this."

In any case, I refused the dapsone, but agreed to a painkiller.

Maritza was getting married that April and I was the maid of honor. The pain I felt was excruciating. The ulcerations blocked the blood flow in my leg. When I stood or walked around, my circulation would push blood through the damaged tissues. My legs felt raw and hot, and the pain was shooting and constant. A few months later, I went to a macrobiotic summer conference in Pennsylvania, where I saw several counselors who recommended that I make plasters out of chlorophyll, aloe vera, brown rice, or sesame oil. I routinely applied a plaster every day for three months, choosing the appropriate one for the healing stage. Eventually the damaged tissue healed from the inside out. The plasters drew the toxins from the tissues of my legs while healing the skin.

After the welts were gone, I went back to my doctor, who was amazed by the healing that had taken place. "How did you do that?" he asked me. "Did you take the medicine I recommended?"

"No," I said. Then I explained the plasters. He just shook his head. My legs still bear the scars that the welts left behind. That was my last health crisis until 1997. Because I had changed my lifestyle to macrobiotics, the surgical graft on my neck had held up well. Through the years, it had been periodically checked. It seems that because I ate well and took care of myself physically, the graft had not deteriorated as quickly as expected. It had not lasted 10 years or less, as the doctors back then had thought, but rather went for 22 years before needing to be replaced. By then, I was in tune with my body and its signals.

The first symptom I felt was heaviness in my neck and shoulders. A few days later, a curtain of shadows seemed to cover my right eye. I knew immediately what was happening. The specialist ordered an artiorgram to determine the extent of the damage. This brought back my old fears of a stroke. It was this particular test that had triggered the stroke when I was 19. However, the specialist reassured me that artiorgrams were more controlled now and that I would be monitored very closely. I knew my physical health was better than it was when I was 19 and that gave me confidence. According to the doctor, my entire carotid artery would have to be replaced with a piece of gortex material because the area in which the Dacron graft had been used could not be patched up again. Gortex is lifetime-durable and used on athletes. The doctor also wanted to replace my aorta with one long piece of gortex because he felt that it would eventually have to be replaced anyway. I quickly refused. I wanted my damaged artery and nothing else replaced. "I have been macrobiotic for seventeen years now, which is why the other graft lasted so long," I explained. "I know my aorta is in perfect shape. Please don't touch it."

My head was spinning as I woke from the anesthesia and I felt a tremendous heaviness in my chest. My mouth and throat were dry when I tried to speak. I had one free hand, which I lifted to my chest and used to feel around for any signs of surgery. The nurse saw me and came over. All I could say was, "Did they cut me here?"

"No," she said, "the surgery was just on your neck." With that, she patted me on the hand and gave me a sip of water. I gave a big sigh of relief, whispered my thanks, and fell back to sleep.

The next day, the doctor agreed that my aorta was in perfect shape and did not need repair. He also said I was recovering quickly and could go home sooner than expected. My recovery at home was peaceful. Eating macrobiotically helped me regain my strength and the incision healed up nicely. I was told that nothing could be done about the partial blockage that remained in my right eye. I would have to adjust to it. I didn't like hearing those words, but I had been told worse news in the past. "We'll see," I responded.

The Healing Continues

That is not to say that the healing has stopped. My illness was the most visible problem I had, certainly the most acute, but below the surface I suffered from many other imbalances, not the least of which was that I hardly knew who I was. When you suffer from a debilitating disease for most of your life, it becomes a part of your identity. It shapes how you think of yourself and who you think you are. The illness defines your immediate limits; it determines, for example, whether you have the energy to get out of bed or leave the house that day. It also limits what you think is possible for your life. Under such circumstances, it's very hard, if not impossible, to know who you are, because your life is trapped behind walls that you cannot see beyond.

I entered adulthood as a woman who believed she did not deserve love, that anyone who did love me would be sacrificing themselves so that I could be happy. That belief was at the bottom of my relationship with Chip. He was the one with the options, the freedom to choose. Not only did I love him, but I was grateful to him for choosing me.

After we were married and fell into our patterns, I believed that my sickness excused Chip from relating to me on a deeper, more intimate level. I was the sick one. I had to be grateful that he would be with me at all. When I got well, however, I naturally awakened to deeper aspects of myself. I found meaning and direction to my life. I wanted to experience life to the fullest. There were no limits now. God had answered my prayers beyond my expectations. I wanted to share those with Chip. I also wanted him to share himself more deeply with me. I wanted us to do all the things that the illness had prevented us from doing as a couple. That wasn't his nature, however. My desire for intimacy served only to drive him farther away from me. In a way, it was easier for him to be with a sick person than it was for him to be with someone healthy.

This, of course, led us into many conflicts. In his frustration, Chip would threaten divorce as a solution. For many months, we saw a marriage counselor for help, but nothing, it seemed, could bring Chip out of his shell. One day, when the counselor was seeing me alone, he asked me if I realized how much I had lost myself in my relationship with Chip.

"What do you mean?" I said.

"You met your husband when you were fifteen years old," he said. "You were young and ill. There's no way you could have known what you needed in a spouse. Your husband is from a reserved Southern Christian family. You are from a passionate

Spanish Christian family. Over the years, you have tried to become more like him, and in the process, you've lost yourself. Your Spanish ancestry is also the basis for much of your femininity, and you've lost that, too. Now you're wondering why things aren't working out and why you're unhappy. It's clear why. You are both very different people, with very different needs."

The counselor's words shocked me—not just because they were so direct and powerful, but because they were so accurate. He summed up my life in a few sentences. I left his office in a state of numb dismay. I didn't know what I was going to do, but I knew that the earth had shifted beneath my feet.

It wasn't long after my meeting with the counselor that Chip took a job in Connecticut, where he lived for a year. That was an informal separation that many years later led to a formal one. We both realized how much we had changed. We knew that our lives had gone in very separate directions and eventually we divorced.

My unfulfilling marriage made me realize that, in my own way, I was running away from my Spanish heritage and from dark, passionate men. In other words, I was running away from my father. I had seen how much my mother had suffered, and on some level, I believed that if I married an unemotional, blond-haired American, I could avoid that kind of suffering. To me, the Harpers were the picture-perfect American family and that's what I thought I wanted. In the end, marrying a man whose emotional expression was very different from my own gave me a new set of problems. Chip had expressed a desire for our family to be warm and loving, like the family I grew up in. But our different expression of "warm and loving" made it difficult for us to realize it.

Almost as soon as I had recovered my health in the spring and summer of 1981, I started to work with a counselor on my relationship with my father. That therapy led me to many realizations about myself, my father and mother, and my husband. Little by little, I came to a greater understanding of my entire family. And then one day, the opportunity to confront my father presented itself.

He became engaged to marry a young woman from Chile

who, in fact, was a beautiful person, though I was hardly ready to recognize that at the time. After they became engaged, my father asked me to attend his wedding. At first, I told him that I wouldn't, that I felt it would be a betrayal of my mother. But he kept asking me until I finally had to tell him how I felt.

We sat together in a quiet room in his house and I explained that when I was a child, I was very confused because I saw my mother and father fighting so much. I saw how much pain my mother was in, especially when my father did not come home at night. He didn't want to be with her. I took that rejection on myself. It seemed that he didn't want to be with either one of us. Since I was the oldest child, I felt that rejection to an even greater extent. Why weren't we good enough for you? I asked him. It seemed that I could do nothing right in his eyes. I grew up feeling somehow flawed and rejected.

I had said all of this in a nonconfrontational way. I was not accusing him so much as explaining what I had experienced and believed.

His reaction was equally soft and understanding. He listened to every word I said without interrupting me or becoming impatient. He just held my words without judging them. When he spoke, he stated his words without anger or blame.

"I always respected your mother, Ginny," my father said. "But we were very different kinds of people. I may not have been a good husband, but I was a good father," he said. "I always tried to be a good father. That was very important to me."

He then proceeded to tell me what he had had to go through as a child and young man and how hard it was for a Chilean who spoke very little English to scratch out a place for himself and his family in this country. Eventually he made a very good living for all of us, but it required him to work very hard and for many long hours. He did not regret any of it and he didn't blame anyone. He was merely doing what he thought was best. But more than anything else in the world, he loved his children and wanted to provide them with the best life he could.

"I love you so much, Ginny," he said. "I always have and always will. I am proud of all my children and they are most important."

As he spoke, a heavy blanket lifted off me. All the conflict, anger, and animosity that had plagued me as a child dissipated. The crying child had finally been heard.

That was my confrontation with my father. I decided to attend his wedding, as did my sister and brother. Eventually, my father and mother reconciled and my mother became a friend to my father's new wife. We were again a big family, though bruised and misshapen. In the end, love had triumphed in its own way.

In the summer of 1986, I fulfilled a promise to myself that had sustained me through a multitude of trials and considerable pain. On a sunny day in June, Chrisi and I rode our bicycles together around our neighborhood. Buddy came along, too, strapped securely in a child's seat on my bicycle. We rode along the green hills under an intimate blue sky. We raced each other, swerved around imaginary obstacles, and laughed with abandon. The image of love and good health, which only seven years earlier seemed like an impossible dream, had become a reality beyond my expectations.

PART TWO

A Program for Overcoming Crohn's and Other IBDs

10

The Digestive System and Enzymes

More than a million Americans suffer from inflammatory bowel disorders, or IBDs. The two most common IBDs are Crohn's, which can afflict both the small and the large intestines, and colitis, which attacks the large intestine or colon. Others include irritable bowel syndrome, a condition that arises from abnormal behavior of the large intestine. There is no evidence of organic disease in irritable bowel syndrome, but there are many severe symptoms, nonetheless. Among them are cramping, pain, gas, bloating, and severe swings between diarrhea and constipation. There is no inflammation associated with the condition and there appears to be no permanent harm to the intestines. The causes include stress and fatty foods, which stimulate the colon to contract and eliminate.

Crohn's and ulcerative colitis are often referred to collectively as inflammatory bowel diseases, which are characterized by inflammation or ulceration in the small and/or the large intestines. The cause or causes are unknown, but medical doctors speculate that they include aberrant genes, a virus or bacteria that penetrates the intestinal wall, and autoimmune reactions that trigger an immune attack against the intestinal tissue. Ulcerative colitis affects the inner lining of the colon and rectum; Crohn's can affect both the small and the large intestines.

Both illnesses tend to spread throughout their respective organs and both arise in people as early as age twelve and as late as age fifty. They are associated with nausea, diarrhea, and severe pain. They can also lead to cancer. People who experience a long-term remission of their IBD, especially for longer than 5 to 7 years, should be checked for colon cancer, to which the IBDs can lead.

Other problems associated with Crohn's include joint pain, fever, loss of appetite, bloody stools, painful stools, abscess, intestinal blockage, infertility, infection, weight loss, and mouth sores.

In Part Two of this book, I want to give you a better understanding of your intestinal tract, teach you about some of the medical options facing you, and then offer a program to combat your IBD. That program includes a healing diet, a variety of natural remedies to promote healing and to deal with a flare-up, lifestyle recommendations that encourage healing, and recipes to help you get started in the kitchen. So let's begin with a better understanding of our intestinal tract, the place where so much suffering can occur.

The Digestive Tract

Our intestines and our lungs are the only two biological systems that receive nourishment from the outer environment. Over the course of 70 years, the intestines process 40 tons of food, digesting it at a rate of about one inch per minute.

The digestive tract is a series of organs joined in a long twisting tube from mouth to anus. That tube is lined with mucosa, or mucus membranes. These membranes are tiny glands that secrete digestive juices when food enters the mouth. Chewing and swallowing assist the process by breaking down the food. As we chew, alkaline saliva helps to break down complex carbohydrates into simple sugars. The saliva also alkalizes the food.

Once food is in our mouths, the brain signals to the stomach that the food is on its way. At that point, the stomach begins secreting digestive juices, including hydrochloric acid (HCL) and pepsin, which assists in the digestion of proteins. The stomach is lined with muscle that churns the food into a soft, liquid mass called chyme. Once it is fully emulsified, the food is passed into the first stage of the small intestine, known as the duodenum.

The small intestine stretches approximately 25 feet—it varies somewhat depending on the individual. The small intestine is lined with millions of hairlike structures called villi, which harbor many types of bacteria. In health, there is a balance between friendly flora and yeast, both of which aid in the breakdown of food and the release of its nutrients.

Enzymes secreted by the pancreas and liver work on the food to make each nutrient available to the bloodstream. The liver also secretes, via the gall bladder, bile acids that break down and emulsify fats and help to absorb the fat-soluble vitamins. Most of the food is absorbed in the small intestine. Water and electrolytes are absorbed in the large intestine, or colon. The lining of the digestive tract contains villi, which separate and sort the nutrients.

There is a vast difference in the way whole, unprocessed foods are digested and absorbed and the way highly refined, or processed, foods are. Whole foods, such as unprocessed grains, vegetables, beans, sea vegetables, and fruit, must be acted on within the small intestine before their nutrients can be absorbed into the bloodstream. All the nutrition and complex carbohydrates in these foods are bound up in their fibrous matrices. The only way to release the nutrition and energy from these foods is for the body to break them down and shower them with enzymes that make the nutrients available to the bloodstream. This is a slow and laborious process. The complex carbohydrates found in these foods are slowly released and slowly absorbed, which is why eating a bowl of brown rice, for example, provides long-lasting energy. The carbohydrates from within that rice are dripped into the bloodstream over many hours, providing long-lasting endurance and energy.

Processed food, such as white flour products, sugar, and foods loaded with artificial ingredients, are rapidly absorbed into the bloodstream. In fact, they do not require digestion at all, but start entering the bloodstream through the mouth and stomach.

This does not give the food a chance to alkalize, which means it contributes to the creation of acidic blood and an acidic environment within the intestinal tract. Acidic blood and digestion are associated with fatigue, as well as many illnesses, including IBDs.

The American diet, of course, provides an abundant supply of artificial ingredients, animal proteins, cholesterol, and fats, all of which contribute to a wide array of illnesses, especially IBD. The American diet is also severely deficient in fiber and plant-based nutrients, antioxidants, and phytochemicals.

A macrobiotic diet is low in fat, cholesterol, and artificial ingredients—it is the intention of the program to eliminate them to the greatest extent possible. At the same time, the diet is rich in phytochemicals, antioxidants, and immune-boosting, cancer-fighting substances. Because it is based on plant foods, the macrobiotic diet is also rich in fiber, which is a source of concern to people with Crohn's and other IBDs. As my story makes clear, and as I explain in detail below, we must reduce the fiber in the macrobiotic diet, at least when first starting the program. We do that by soaking grains and beans overnight, cooking with more water, and using a food mill to grind the food into a soft, low-fiber mass. The resulting food soothes and heals the intestinal tract, while providing optimal nutrition.

The macrobiotic view on Crohn's, ulcerative colitis, and other IBDs is that they arise from the consumption of a high-acid, low-fiber diet. The acidic condition arises for several reasons. First, protein is converted to uric acid during digestion. The higher the protein content of your diet, the higher your acid levels will be. This is the very reason, as any knowledgeable doctor or researcher will tell you, a high-protein diet is associated with higher levels of osteoporosis. The body must buffer, or alkalize, the high acid levels caused by the high-protein diet by leaching calcium and phosphorous from the bones. In emergency situations, such as high acid levels, those minerals are the body's natural alkalizing agents. Unfortunately, it's like burning the furniture and wood in your house to stay warm: eventually, your house collapses, just as the body does when the bones become osteoporotic.

Other substances elevate the acid levels, as well. They include processed sugars, artificial ingredients, and refined white flour.

As the acid levels increase, healthy intestinal flora are destroyed. Replacing that flora are bacteria that themselves produce acidic substances, as well as estrogen-like compounds. Increasingly, illness-producing bacteria and viruses take up residence within the intestinal tract. The net result is that the intestinal tract becomes increasingly acidic and unhealthy. The body attempts to protect itself against these conditions by making the intestinal walls thick and inflamed. Not only do we experience malabsorption, but also symptoms begin one by one. All of these conditions combine to create sores and ulcers, which lead to more inflammation and, eventually, to a disease state such as Crohn's or ulcerative colitis. Long before the illness sets in, the signs and symptoms ("body signals," as I call them) were there, but the person did not know how to change the conditions that would alleviate the problem.

IBDs are diagnosed through physical examination, blood tests, upper and lower GI examinations, colonoscopy, and biopsy. All of these show the diseased state of the digestive tract.

Understanding balance, or the state of "ease," for health is important. "Dis-ease" is not evil, but the body's natural attempt to survive and to return to a state that is dynamic and harmonious with its surroundings. Macrobiotics looks at the root cause of disease—the where, how, why, and when. It addresses not only how we nourish our bodies, but also the environmental stresses on them.

By learning the natural law of nature that for every action there is a reaction, we can view ourselves and our bodies the way God intended: We are not victims of circumstance, but responsible stewards of the temples we were given. When our bodies are out of balance, they are more sensitive to change and more susceptible to illness.

The medical community addresses symptoms, not causes, and

therefore is limited in its attempts to achieve total recovery. More and more people today are realizing the futility of seeking just symptom relief. The biggest challenge of society today is twofold. First, we must overcome our ignorance regarding the simple yet profound truth that what we eat and how we live impact and shape our lives. Second, we must conquer our shortsighted desire for quick, magical cures.

Just as life always tends toward resolutions, so does the physical body tend toward health.

Enzymes: Essential Chemicals for Healthy Digestion

Enzymes, or chemical catalysts produced by the body, are responsible for the normal function of every organ and system, including both the immune and digestive systems. Many biochemists refer to enzymes as "the life energy" of all organisms. Without an adequate supply of enzymes, the digestion and assimilation of nutrients is significantly impaired, as are the functioning of the other organs and systems.

Enzymes are produced by the body but are also present in food. We are born with a limited supply of enzymes and can produce only a finite number during our lifetime. This is important to intestinal health because digestion is always given precedence over the other bodily functions. If the body's enzyme production is low and the diet doesn't include enough foods rich in enzymes, the body will draw the enzymes it needs for digestion away from the other bodily functions. The result is a body with a lowered disease-fighting capability and a general weakening of the ability to regenerate. Supplying the body with high-quality, enzyme-rich foods will prevent this enzyme shortage from occurring. The more whole and unprocessed the food, the richer it is in enzymes. Raw foods contain more enzymes than cooked foods, because many enzymes are lost during cooking. The problem for people with IBD, of course, is that they cannot tolerate raw foods, at least until the health of their digestive system improves, which means they must get their enzymes from other sources, which I address below. Processed foods are markedly deficient in enzymes, a condition that shifts the burden for supplying enzymes on the body.

A healthy enzymatic environment within the digestive tract is crucial for the proper metabolism, absorption, and assimilation of nutrients. Indeed, these powerful chemicals help keep us alive. There are more than 3,000 known enzymes that are essential for as many bodily functions. Enzymes help to convert the food we eat into both potential and kinetic energy. The work of such conversion is masterminded by genes within our cells.

Enzymes are highly sensitive substances. They are easily damaged or destroyed by excess heat, microwaves, refining, pasteurization, smoking, various forms of pollution, excessive exposure to sunlight, radiation, and drugs. Without sufficient digestive enzymes, numerous glands within our endocrine system—including the thyroid gland—fail to function properly. As we age, our exposure to pollution, cigarette smoke, microwaves, refined foods, pasteurization, and other insults increases, which means our total enzyme supply, as well as our capacity to produce enzymes, diminishes. This is particularly crucial to people with IBD, because enzymes are essential for restoring a healthy digestive system. If the ability to absorb nutrients through the intestinal wall into the bloodstream is disturbed, the whole digestive system ceases to function. The result is gastrointestinal discomfort.

The three most important enzymes for the digestive tract are amylase, protease, and lipase.

Amylase is secreted in the mouth and is an essential ingredient in saliva. It initiates the digestion of carbohydrates, thus making them more absorbable within the small intestine. Amylase continues to convert carbohydrates into absorbable compounds in the duodenum at a rate of about 300 grams of carbohydrate per hour.

Protease, which is activated by the hydrochloric acid in the stomach, breaks down up to 300 grams of protein per hour. The stomach produces one to two liters of gastric juices daily containing, primarily, hydrochloric acid and two helper enzymes—pepsin and cathepsin.

Lipase breaks down 175 grams of fat per hour. Fat is initially acted upon by bile acids—secreted by the gall bladder—which convert it to a solution. It is then acted upon by the lipase.

All three of these enzymes are essential for healthy digestion. Without adequate supplies of them, digestion is weakened and the body is extremely vulnerable to disease. Inadequate supplies of amylase have been shown to give rise to allergies, fatigue, inflammation, and irritable bowel syndrome; low supplies of protease contribute to constipation, parasites, and IBS. Inadequate lipase is associated with disorders of the gall bladder, increased stress, constipation, diarrhea, and IBS.

Replacing Essential Enzymes

Virtually all adults in modern America suffer from insufficient enzyme supplies and would benefit by taking supplemental enzymes, but supplementation is essential for people with IBD. Enzyme supplements come in pills and capsules. For people whose stomachs react to pills, I recommend using the capsules, either by swallowing them as part of a meal or opening them and pouring their contents onto food. Enzymes are activated the minute they touch water, so it's important to eat the food soon after sprinkling on the enzymes.

I recommend supplementing with all three of these digestive enzymes: amylase, protease, and lipase. All three should be taken three times a day, at each meal. Once symptoms diminish, then you can cut back. It is appropriate to take an enzyme before a large meal regardless. Take the following quantities:

Amylase—10,000 international units (IU)
Protease—30,000 international units
Lipase—145 international units

Very important: Make sure that the digestive enzymes you take are plant-based, meaning they originate from plant sources. Plant-based nutrients are safe, effective, and easily assimilated by the body.

Replenishing your digestive system with health-promoting enzymes is an essential step in the healing process. But the overall health of your digestive system is determined by what you eat. The right diet can heal you of Crohn's disease, ulcerative colitis, and other IBDs. That healing program is described in the next chapter.

11

A Program to Heal Crohn's and Other IBDs

The goal of the macrobiotic diet is to heal the intestinal tract of all existing IBDs. Strictly speaking, macrobiotics creates the appropriate conditions for the body to heal itself. It does this by changing the intestinal environment in several ways, including the following:

- It reduces the overall acidity in the intestines and makes the environment more alkaline.
- It increases the amount of friendly, health-promoting flora.
- It increases the amount of digestive enzymes.
- It increases the amount of immune-boosting, cancer-fighting vitamins, minerals, and phytochemicals, which are abundant in plant-based foods and promote healing.
- It decreases the amount of illness-promoting flora.
- It reduces parasites within the intestines.
- It reduces or eliminates the food substances that contribute to inflammation, such as dairy products and sugars.
- It reduces or eliminates artificial ingredients and toxic substances, which are present in processed foods.

One of the most difficult challenges we face is finding and sustaining a health-promoting diet.

When I first began my healing diet, I saw food within a very narrow framework—that is, how it affected me physically. I saw the diet as a prescription for getting well. There were "right" foods and "wrong" foods. At the beginning of our attempts to heal ourselves, this is an inescapable and appropriate way to see things. But as your health improves and your intestinal strength returns, your flexibility increases. There will always be foods that you are better off avoiding entirely, but your capacity to enjoy a wider variety of foods increases dramatically, as your health returns. This means that when you begin the diet, you should be as strict as possible to get the maximum benefit from the program. After your health has improved, you can begin to widen your eating habits.

Here is a step-by-step approach to transforming your way of eating to one that can, if followed correctly, help you recover from Crohn's, ulcerative colitis, or any other IBD.

Step One: Discontinue All Refined Products and Processed Foods

I am talking about anything white. This means any food item that is in a can, package, or wrapper, or that is frozen. These types of food usually have long ingredient lists of unpronounceable words. Most have been denatured, which means that they have been stripped of their nutrients and then had some selected vitamins or minerals put back. Such foods often contain high quantities of preservatives, colors, and flavors.

Step Two: Discontinue All Processed and Refined Sugars

Processed and refined sugars include white table sugar, brown sugar, honey, molasses, fructose, sucrose, dextrose, corn syrup, corn solids, juice concentrate, and malt. Sugars rob the body of minerals and stimulate inflammatory cytokines, or chemical messengers within the immune system that promote inflammation. They also dramatically increase acidity within the intestinal tract.

Step Three: Discontinue All Dairy Products

Stop consuming all cow's milk and products from cow's milk, including butter, skim milk, 1 percent milk, yogurt, and mayonnaise. Cow's milk is vastly different from human milk in a number of essential ways. Cow's milk is acidic, while human milk is alkaline. Human milk helps strengthen the baby's immune system, making the child more resistant to disease for the rest of his or her life. Human milk also promotes the growth of the human nervous system, including the brain. It makes the child better able to digest cholesterol and provides an abundance of health-promoting bacteria. Cow's milk provides lots of calcium and protein, essentially because it is intended to help a calf rapidly develop bone structure and physical girth. The proteins in cow's milk, trigger an immune reaction in sensitive children, thus causing the body's defenses to attack healthy tissue. Finally, most humans lose the ability to produce lactase, the enzyme needed to digest milk sugar, or lactose, as they mature. As that enzyme diminishes in quantity and eventually is lost, the body suffers an array of symptoms—including bloating, belching, gas, acidic bowels, constipation and diarrhea—whenever milk products are consumed.

Milk products provide an array of toxins and proteins that trigger autoimmune reactions against the body. Three substances stand out as particularly deleterious: milk sugar, milk fat, and milk protein. Let's look at these individually.

Milk Sugar

The sugar in cow's milk is called lactose, which is formed from two simple sugars, glucose and galactose. When the amount of lactose exceeds the body's ability to break it down or utilize it, bacteria in the intestinal tract act upon the lactose to produce gas, carbon dioxide, and lactic acid. These substances then combine with water to create bloating, indigestion, and cramping. Typically, humans lose some or all of their ability to digest lactose in their youth, which makes all of these problems more likely. Lactose activity first appears before birth, during the third trimester of gestation. It gradually diminishes between the ages of one and a half and four years. For some people, the problems caused by this "lactose intolerance" can become more severe.

Milk Fat

A quart of milk contains 35 grams of fat, with 60 percent of whole milk being saturated fat. These 35 grams represent about half of all the fat an average 150-pound man should consume in one day.

Fat is a leading cause of coronary heart disease, many common forms of cancer—including those of the colon, breast, and prostate—and adult-onset diabetes. Saturated fat stimulates the liver to make more cholesterol. High cholesterol leads to atherosclerosis, which is a buildup of plaque in the arterial vessels. Atherosclerosis is a slow process that generally takes close to 20 years to develop. The plaques that line the arterial walls in atherosclerosis are rich in fat, due to cholesterol. Atherosclerosis can lead to vessel obstruction or coronary disease, which can result in stroke or heart attack.

Milk Protein

A landmark study published in *The New England Journal of Medicine* in July 1992 revealed that cow's milk can stimulate an autoimmune reaction against the human pancreas and give rise to juvenile diabetes in sensitive children.

Scientists discovered that children produce antibodies when their systems are confronted with the proteins in cow's milk, specifically bovine albumin peptide. The cow's milk proteins attach themselves to the surface of the pancreas, the organ that produces insulin. Insulin is the hormone used by the body to make sugar available to the cells. Without insulin, the cells die. When the antibodies attack the cow's milk proteins, they very likely destroy the insulin-producing beta cells of the pancreas, as well. This, of course, destroys the pancreas's ability to produce insulin.

Scientists have known for many years that childhood diabetes is caused by an immune response that destroys the insulin-producing cells. Animal studies have shown that cow's milk can trigger that autoimmune reaction and cause diabetes. Moreover, researchers have found that diabetes turns up in wealthy populations that consume large quantities of dairy products. Conversely, it has been found to be rare in populations that do not consume cow's milk, such as Asians and Africans. Researchers have also found that feeding infants only breast milk not only delays the consumption of milk products, but also reduces the risk of childhood diabetes.

Other studies have shown that dairy products are linked with an increase in inflammatory arthritis, which is far more common in the dairy-consuming Western nations, such as the United States, Canada, Europe, Australia, and New Zealand, than in other parts of the world.

One of the primary causes of arthritis is an immune reaction caused by the presence of animal proteins in the blood, especially the proteins from dairy foods. Once animal proteins make their way into the blood of sensitive people, the immune system produces antibodies whose mission is to attack and destroy these proteins. The proteins combine with the antibodies to form compounds called "immune complexes." The immune complexes take up residence in the joints and act as irritants, much the same way a sliver of wood would irritate your tissues if it were placed in one or more of your joints.

Dairy products are acid-producing, especially in the digestive tract. They contribute to a host of illnesses, not the least of which is IBD. Cow's milk is acidic, while human milk is alkaline. When a human mother nurses her baby, she transfers her immunization against many diseases to her baby. She also gives her baby a lifetime supply of the intestinal bacteria and flora needed for health. A baby calf weighs about 130 pounds when it's born. One month later, it weighs about 240 pounds. This is why cow's milk contains so much calcium. Calves need lots of calcium to grow physically. Human milk contains more phosphorus than calcium. Phosphorus is very important for brain growth and development. In human babies, the brain develops first, while in animal babies, bone structure develops first.

Is it any wonder we have over-grown, overweight children who are developing faster and bigger with each generation? Our children now suffer with asthma, allergies, attention deficit disorder (ADD), attention deficit-hyperactivity disorder (ADHD), bronchitis, chest infection, acne, anemia, bloated abdomen, cramps, constipation, diabetes, diarrhea, eczema, gastrointestinal disturbances, and hay fever, just to name a few ailments. All this because we bought into the slogan, "Milk—it does a body good."

Step Four: Discontinue All Red Meat, Pork, and Chicken

To eat meat, you have to cook it, often at high heat to avoid the *E. coli* and other bacterial problems associated with meat consumption. But the higher the heat, the more the digestive enzymes are lost, which means the meat becomes more difficult to digest. Also, high heat changes the ionic bonds within the fat molecules, making them more toxic within human tissue, primarily because they break down more rapidly, become rancid, and form free radicals. Free radicals, also known as oxidants, are the primary source of more than 60 illnesses, including heart disease, cancer, arthritis, immune depression, and a variety of IBDs. Meat is a very big producer of free radicals.

Meat consumption gives rise to high levels of acid within the intestines, thanks to the protein and fat.

Meat consumption is associated with significantly higher rates of heart disease, cancer, adult-onset diabetes, high blood pressure, osteoporosis, and a wide array of digestive disorders.

The truth is, humans have great difficulty fully masticating and digesting a piece of beef or pork, for example. The reason is that we are poorly equipped physiologically to handle the tough, sinuous meat. Thus, our physiological design gives us only a limited capacity to eat the various forms of meat, especially the tough meats such as beef, pork, and chicken.

Carnivores have a very simple and short digestive system—usually about three times the length of their bodies. This permits the rapid expulsion of putrefactive bacteria and the decomposing flesh. Flesh decays very rapidly and the by-products quickly become toxic in the bloodstream. They are especially poisonous if they remain there for any length of time. Carnivores also have acidic saliva, unlike humans, who have alkaline saliva.

The stomachs of carnivores also have ten times as much hydrochloric acid as the stomachs of herbivores to digest tough, sinuous tissues and bones.

Noncarnivorous animals, such as human beings, have long digestive tracts—usually about twelve times the length of their bodies. Their saliva contains ptyalin for predigesting of grains. Their stomach acids are one-twentieth as acidic as those of meat eaters. Their intestines are alkaline to absorb nutrients and separate waste.

Many people would be shocked to discover that today's animal products are very different from those of our grandparents, whose animals roamed freely on the farm. They killed only what they needed at the time for their meal. Growing up on a chicken farm in Chile, I used to help my grandmother catch the chicken. She would twist its neck and kill it instantly. She would cook and use every part of it. She would even boil down the bones to make chicken stock. But the animal foods would be only a part of our meal. The rest would be vegetables.

Today, animals are routinely fed hormones to make them grow faster, bigger, and fatter. They are given antibiotics to prevent disease. Even the way they are slaughtered today should give one pause. It is horribly cruel and inhumane. The experience of the fear leading up to the slaughter and the actual death itself remains in the tissues of the animal in the form of hormones, known as pheromones, which people consume as part of their food. Other chemical changes occur before and during the slaughter, including increases in uric acid, adrenaline, and other toxic wastes, which remain in the blood and tissue. These poisons then get stuck in our tissues. And then there is the question of how much bacteria is present in the meat by the time it arrives on our dinner plate.

Meat passes very slowly through the human digestive system, taking about five days to be fully eliminated. Vegetable foods take about a day and a half. The longer undigested meat remains in the digestive tract, the more the toxins within the meat—such as the fat and preservatives—can act on our small and large intestine. Sodium nitrite, a common preservative and chemical used to cure meats, for example, gives rise to nitrous acid, which becomes a carcinogen when mixed with our stomach acids. The reactions to this and other chemicals found in meat include acid reflux, indigestion, burning, bloating, diarrhea, and nausea. Sharp pain and weakened digestion can also occur.

Step Five: Discontinue All Flour Products

Wheat is among the most difficult grains to digest. It is very hard and fibrous. The wheat fiber also has a damaging effect on the tips of the villi, the fingerlike projections within the small intestine that absorb the nutrients. When exposed to significant amounts of wheat, the villi tend to shrink. Gluten increases the mucous content of the intestines, making them sluggish and acidic. Be careful of breads containing rye, barley, and oats, all of which have a high gluten content. They can cause constipation and other forms of indigestion.

Step Six:. Discontinue All Cold Drinks, Sugared Drinks, Carbonated Sodas, Juices, and Tap Water

Avoid vegetable and fruit juices and stimulant teas, iced or hot. These drinks slow down and paralyze the digestive processes and irritate the intestinal lining. (Soda pop is sometimes used to clean car battery terminals! It is very acidic and corrosive.)

Drink spring water. The recommended daily amount is half your body weight in ounces. If you weigh 100 pounds, your recommended water allotment is 50 ounces, or about six 8 ounce glasses of water per day. Keep in mind, however, that the food you will be eating is loaded with water. Especially at the beginning of the program, you will be adding extra water to your cooking to make your food soft and easily digestible. When you drink, be conscious of your body's reaction to the water. Are you craving the water? If so, drink more frequently. If your body is getting enough water, you will not be experiencing much thirst.

Avoid drinking highly chemicalized city water. It's not unusual for a city to add 26 or more chemical ingredients to water. Many of them are dubious and some are clearly toxic to human health.

Distilled water is condensed vapor. It does not have minerals. Drinking it on a regular basis will leach essential minerals from the body.

Step Seven: Discontinue the Use of all Chemicals and Pollutants

As much as possible, eat only organically grown vegetables and fruits. Prior to World War II, few chemical herbicides, insecticides, and fertilizers were used in U.S. agriculture. After the food was harvested, even fewer chemicals were added to the food. It wasn't colored, sweetened, or preserved nearly as much as it is today.

When our bodies take in a non-food item, they don't know what to do with it. If they can't break it down with strong acids and eliminate it, they will store it somewhere in the body to deal with later, maybe even years later. Toxic chemicals are stored in the fat cells and lymph glands. They remain in the body for decades. They make the body weak and unable to combat illness. These stored substances create weakness in the immune system, congestion in the organs, and plaque in the intestines.

In the 1950s and 1960s, the toxins used by farmers were more topical and could be peeled or washed off the vegetable after it was purchased. Today, however, the poisons are so strong that they are metabolized by the plant and thus become an integral part of it. There's no way you can escape some of these poisons if you eat food that has been treated with them.

Therefore, I recommend that you eat as much organically grown food as possible and avoid all artificial ingredients, such as colors, flavors, and preservatives.

Here are just a few of the more commonly used chemicals in foods to watch for:

- *Acesulfamek.* A sugar substitute sold as Sunette and Sweet One. Acesulfamek has a chemical structure similar to that of saccharin. It is known to cause cancer in animals.
- *Artificial colorings.* Chemicals that add color to food. Derived from coal tar these synthetic dyes have only one purpose— to make food prettier and thus sell better. The FDA has banned 13 synthetic food colorants since 1956 because of health concerns. The two that still remain are red number 3 and yellow number 5, both of which are linked to thyroid cancer in lab rats.
- *Aspartame.* A sugar substitute sold as Equal and Nutrasweet. The FDA has approved the use of aspartame in all foods, including food that does not require labeling, such as fast food. However, the U.S. Air Force has warned its pilots not to drink diet soft drinks sweetened with aspartame before flying because they have been associated with grand mal seizures in commercial pilots.
- *Butylated hydroxyanisole and butylated hydroxytoluene (BHA and BHT).* Synthetic preservatives designed to prevent oxidation and retard rancidity. They are added to foods that contain oil and to dry cereals. A 1982 study showed that BHA affected the growth hormones in rats.
- *Monosodium glutamate (MSG).* A flavor-enhancing amino acid. Only half of this amino acid is acceptable, however. Glutamate is a naturally occurring amino acid found in car-

rots and whole grains that is essential for human health. However, when it is combined with monosodium, it becomes toxic, especially when consumed in large quantities. MSG can cause the neurons in the brain to become over-stimulated and die. A side effect of this event is headaches. MSG is disguised on processed food labels as textured vegetable protein (TVP) or plant protein extract. Also called "hydrolyzed," it is added to frozen foods to help them retain their flavor. Common side effects are lightness in the chest, drowsiness, headaches, burning sensations in the forearms and on the back of the neck, and burning and cramping in the stomach.

- *Olestra.* A synthetic or "fake" fat. It was approved by the FDA for use in snack foods, despite the objections registered by numerous scientists. Olestra can become attached to valuable nutrients in the body and promote their elimination. The Harvard School of Public Health states that olestra causes diarrhea and other gastrointestinal problems, even at low doses. It has also been known to cause anal leakage, cramping, and loose stools. According to the FDA, all foods that contain olestra must be labeled with a warning. In other words, it's essential that you read labels.

- *Recombinant bovine growth hormone (rBGH).* A genetically engineered drug that is injected into dairy cows to increase their milk production. Residues of the drug are passed on to humans in the cows' milk. To compound the problem, rBGH cause disease in the cows. The cows are then given antibiotics, which are also passed on in their milk.

- *Sulfites.* Synthetically produced chemicals that prevent discoloration, bacterial growth, and fermentation of vegetables. They are used most often to keep foods looking fresh after they have been cut. Sulfites can provoke severe allergic reactions, including asthma. In 1985 the FDA linked at least 12 asthma-related deaths to sulfites. The FDA banned use of the substance on most fruits and vegetables, except in fresh-cut potatoes, dried fruit, and wine. Don't buy nonorganic vegetables that look perfect. They may have harmful, synthetic ingredients to thank for their good looks.

In addition, avoid over-the-counter medications and prescription drugs that can adversely affect intestinal health. Among them are aspirin, ibuprofen, and antibiotics. Also avoid nicotine, excessive alcohol, and meat tenderizers.

Step Eight: Begin a Standard Macrobiotic Diet

There is no "one" macrobiotic diet. There are many variations of the program, depending on your needs, symptoms, condition, age, and digestive health. In general, the macrobiotic diet is composed of about 40 to 50 percent whole, unprocessed grains, such as brown rice, barley, millet, buckwheat, wheat, oats, and corn. Approximately 30 to 40 percent of the diet is composed of vegetables, 10 percent of beans and sea vegetables, and about 10 percent of soups, fish, condiments, fruit, and various desserts. As much as possible, try to make sure your foods are grown organically, without the use of artificial pesticides, fertilizers or herbicides.

The staple food of macrobiotics, of course, is whole, unprocessed grains. Let's begin by looking at the grains and grain dishes. (For preparation instructions for these foods, see Chapter 12.)

Whole Grains

Whole grains are an essential for all people working to reestablish good health, but they are especially vital to people with IBD. Between 40 and 50 percent of each meal should be composed of whole grains.

For people with IBD, grains should be prepared with an abundance of water. When boiling, use 5 to 6 cups of water for every cup of grain. If the grain still contains too much fiber, run it through a hand-turned food mill (such as a Foley food mill), which will strain the grain and remove most of the fiber. The creamed grain will be better accepted and easier to digest. Pre-soaking, cooking, and thorough chewing dramatically improve the digestibility of grains.

People with Crohn's, ulcerative colitis, or another intestinal disorder should use only brown rice and millet. Both are soft-shelled grains and the best grains to eat on a daily basis. Brown rice and millet can be soaked for as little as 25 minutes to an hour, and for as long as overnight. Soaking makes them more digestible. Introduce the other grains only when intestinal health has been restored.

When pressure-cooking, use 1½ cups of water for every cup of pre-soaked grain. Use 2–3 cups of water for every cup of grain that has not been presoaked.

Pressure-cooking is good for people who are in a weakened condition and not used to eating grains. The total cooking time for presoaked grain should be 50 minutes. Otherwise, allow 1 hour of total cooking time.

Whole grains are high in vitamin B and have six of the major amino acids. Grains are acid-forming in their natural state, but when cooked with a pinch of sea salt and chewed thoroughly, they become alkaline in the body.

Among the whole grains are the following:

- *Amaranth.* Higher in protein and calcium than milk, amaranth is also higher in the calcium supporting cofactors magnesium and silicon. It is an especially helpful food for pregnant or nursing women, infants, children, people who do heavy physical labor, and people who want to gain weight. Amaranth is a cooling and astringent food. It is used traditionally to strengthen the lungs. It controls bleeding and helps check diarrhea and excessive menstruation. Amaranth becomes sticky when cooked.
- *Brown rice,* including short-, medium-, long-grain brown and basmati. Rice has long been used for intestinal health. It also elevates the level of serotonin, a chemical neurotrans-

mitter that increases the sense of well-being, optimism, and the ability to concentrate.

Whole grain brown rice is the best food for daily consumption. It is the grain with the widest array of nutrients and the easiest to digest. It is beneficial for the nervous system and the brain, and supports colon activity. It is especially healing for people with IBD. The germ of brown rice contains phosphorus, which helps expel toxins from the body.

In addition to standard brown rice, there is also sweet brown rice, which is more glutinous. People with IBD should be careful about the gluten in sweet rice. Note any reactions you may have to it and, if necessary, avoid it in favor of standard brown rice.

- *Buckwheat.* Also known as kasha, buckwheat can be eaten as noodles, as a cereal, or as a stuffing for cabbage or green peppers in place of meat. It is excellent in cold and humid weather since it produces heat quickly. If eaten in warm weather, it should be taken in the evening.

  Buckwheat is high in vitamin E and is traditionally used to strengthen the kidneys. It is best mixed with a vegetable, such as cabbage, or a soft cooking grain, such as millet or quinoa.

- *Corn.* Dried corn meal and flour are very health-promoting when used as polenta and combined with beans. Fresh corn on the cob is a good cooling grain for hot weather. Corn is the sweetest grain and has long been used to strengthen the heart and small intestine. Introduce corn slowly and in creamed form at first.

- *Millet.* The only alkaline grain, millet is excellent for people with acidosis or bad breath. It is high in protein. Millet croquettes are a balanced and delicious food. (For a recipe, see Chapter 13.) Millet supports the spleen-pancreas function and is healing for the digestive tract. After rice, it should be the grain most frequently eaten.

- *Pearled barley,* or hulled barley. The most digestible form of barley, pearled barley is delicious when cooked in soups or served with vegetables. Barley flakes can be made into an excellent morning cereal. Barley is beneficial for breaking up mucus in the body.

After rice, barley is the easiest grain to digest. Because barley is high in gluten, it should be cooked with other grains, such as brown rice, to reduce the amount of gluten consumed. Barley is used traditionally to break up masses and eliminate mucus from the intestines.

- *Quinoa.* This high-energy grain is easily digestible and has a light, nutty flavor. Higher in protein than most other grains, it provides great endurance. Traditionally, it is considered to be drying and warming, as well as strengthening to the kidneys and heart. The grain expands to four times its volume when cooked.

- *Rye.* Excellent as an ingredient in breads and morning cereals, rye is similar to wheat but lower in gluten. For people with IBD, rye should be introduced late in the healing process because it is very high in fiber.

- *Spelt.* This ancient red wheat has a delicious light and nutty flavor. It contains 30 percent more protein than hard red wheat and considerable B vitamins, magnesium, and fiber. It can be easily substituted for wheat in recipes and is well tolerated by many wheat-sensitive people. When soaking spelt, use 3 cups of water for every cup of grain.

- *Teff.* So small that 150 grains weigh the same as a single kernel of wheat, teff has a sweet flavor and a high mineral content. It is a rich source of calcium, magnesium, boron, copper, phosphorus, and zinc. It also contains twice as much iron as wheat and barley. It is gluten-free. Traditionally, teff has been used to support the kidneys, stomach, and spleen-pancreas. It is great for thickening soups.

- *Whole oats.* Make your oatmeal either from fresh steel-cut oats or whole oats, which can be cooked overnight. Oat flakes or rolled oats are highly refined and should not be considered a staple food. They are wonderful, however, in soups and cookies. Oats are high in fat and have been used traditionally for people with sluggish thyroid glands. Those people who have much stored protein tolerate oatmeal much better than rice or buckwheat cream.

- *Whole wheat berries.* Wheat can be made into morning cereals and pancakes, as well as into other products such as noodles, bulghur, and couscous. Wheat is the grain with the highest protein and gluten content. Traditionally, it has been used to treat and heal the liver.

For people with IBD, wheat is the last grain that should be introduced into the diet and should be used only after intestinal health has been firmly reestablished.

Vegetables

Vegetables, the best weapons against disease, should compose between 40 and 60 percent of your daily diet. They not only provide an abundance of vitamins, minerals, and phytochemicals, but they detoxify the body. Their fiber, enzymes, phytonutrients, and antioxidants make them powerful allies in both the prevention and the treatment of disease.

Vegetables should be cooked before eaten. Your symptoms should determine how thoroughly to cook them. If you have not been eating vegetables, introduce them slowly, in small amounts, and only after you have boiled them until very soft. You will not cook away all their nutrients. Boiling reduces the nutrient content of vegetables slightly, but it is more important at this point to retrain your intestines to accept the veggies.

Begin with the round and root vegetables. Cook them in small amounts of water with a pinch of salt. Low boil or steam them for 7 to10 minutes. For sensitive digestion cook them for 15 to 20 minutes, then mash them with a fork using the cooking water. The intestines easily accept creamed vegetables. Introduce the leafy greens only when your symptoms of diarrhea have stopped. The leafy greens are very fibrous and stimulate elimination. To aid the digestion of all these vegetables even more, add a two-inch-square piece of the sea vegetable kombu while cooking the vegetable. The mineral content of the kombu will alkalinize and tenderize the vegetable and aid in its digestion.

Root Vegetables

Traditionally, root vegetables are used to treat the digestive system, particularly the intestines. Roots are the intestines of the plant, since they absorb the nutrients from the soil and distribute them to the plant's circulatory system. The human intestines, of course, do the same thing: They draw the nutrients from the products of the soil, namely the plant and animal foods, and make those nutrients available to the circulatory system.

Root vegetables, therefore, have long been seen as healing for both the small and the large intestines. They are rich in nutrition, especially antioxidants, vitamins, and minerals. The best root vegetables to eat often are carrot, burdock, parsnip, and daikon. Daikon aids in the digestion of whole grains and vegetables. It also helps eliminate excess water and animal fats from the body and has a variety of other medicinal uses.

Root vegetables that can be consumed on a daily basis include:

Burdock	Lotus root
Carrot	Parsnip
Daikon radish	Red radish
Dandelion root	Rutabaga
Jinenjo	Turnip

Round Vegetables

Traditionally, sweet vegetables such as squash were seen as healing to the spleen, stomach, and pancreas. In Chinese medicine, the spleen is considered the governor of digestion because it is the distributor of the life energy, or *Qi*, to the stomach and small and large intestines. The round vegetables provide natural digestible sugars that help relax the body and any contracted organs. The liver and large intestine benefit from both raw and cooked round vegetables. These vegetables are very tasty and soothing to the intestines when creamed.

Round vegetables that can be consumed on a daily basis include:

Acorn squash	Hokkaido pumpkin
Brussels sprouts	Hubbard squash
Buttercup squash	Onion
Butternut squash	Pumpkin
Cabbage	Rutabaga
Cauliflower	Turnip

Leafy Greens

Leafy green vegetables are among the most abundant sources of antioxidants, phytochemicals, vitamins, and minerals on the planet. They are an indispensable source of chlorophyll, which helps create healthy red blood cells. These cells carry oxygen throughout the body. During healing, the oxygen demands are increased, which is one of the many reasons leafy green vegetables are essential to the healing process.

Leafy green vegetables can be steamed, boiled, or blanched. When the level of intestinal sensitivity is high, they should be cooked thoroughly and used in small amounts. As intestinal activity settles and digestion becomes more normalized and stronger, adjust the cooking times and amounts accordingly. Ultimately, you should eat lightly steamed greens three times a day.

The leafy greens that can be consumed on a daily basis include:

Bok choy	Mizuma
Broccoli	Mustard greens
Carrot tops	Parsley
Chinese cabbage	Scallions
Collard greens	String beans
Dandelion greens	Turnip tops
Kale	Watercress
Leeks	

Occasional Vegetables

In addition to the root vegetables, round vegetables, and leafy greens that can be consumed on a daily basis, there are a number of vegetables that can be consumed once or twice a week. These vegetables that can be consumed occasionally include:

Celery	Mushrooms
Chives	Pattypan squash
Coltsfoot	Red cabbage
Cucumber	Romaine lettuce
Endive	Salsify
Escarole	Shiitake mushrooms
Green peas	Snap peas
Iceberg lettuce	Snow peas
Jerusalem artichoke	Sprouts
Kohlrabi	Summer squash
Lambsquarter	Wax beans

The Nightshades

The only group of vegetables you should avoid, especially when your IBD symptoms are active, are the nightshades, which are highly acidic and astringent. The nightshades contain high levels of oxalic acid and solanine. When these acids accumulate in the body, they weaken the intestines and increase pain and inflammation. The nightshades deplete the body of calcium, other minerals, and trace elements, which contributes to, or can trigger, an intestinal crisis.

Rheumatoid arthritis can be much relieved by avoiding these vegetables, tomatoes in particular. When first introduced to Europe, tomatoes were thought to be a deadly poison. Today, their vines and suckers are known to be poisonous to livestock. White potatoes contain solanine, which depletes the body of calcium; therefore, they contribute to nervousness and sleeplessness.

The nightshades cause irritation and inflammation in the intestinal tract. They should be introduced back into the diet only when intestinal health has been fully restored. Once they are reintroduced, they should be eaten only in small portions compared to the other vegetables.

The nightshades include:

Artichoke
Asparagus
Avocado
Bamboo shoots
Beet
Curly dock
Eggplant
Erns Ginseng
Fennel
New Zealand spinach
Okra
Peppers (green and red)

Plantain
Potato
Purslane
Shepherd's purse
Sorrel
Spinach
Sweet potato
Swiss chard
Tomato
Yams
Zucchini

Sea Vegetables

There is no greater source of minerals, vitamins, and phyto-chemicals on earth than sea vegetables. Sea vegetables—especially hijiki, kombu, and wakame—also contain sodium alginate, which scientists at McGill University in Canada have found neutralize and help eliminate radioactive particles and heavy metals from the body. Sea vegetables are concentrated foods. You need to eat only small amounts of them—1 to 2 tablespoons per serving—to derive their enormous benefits. Over 75 species of sea vegetables are eaten around the world.

You can presoak seaweed or cut it up and use it in soups, as a vegetable, or in other dishes. Following are the varieties, their unique qualities, and cooking suggestions:

- *Agar-agar.* These crystal slices of algae are used as a thickener and base in custards, Jell-O, aspic, and mousses. Agar-agar is a natural gelatin, best used in flake form. The flakes have no taste or aroma. They simply need to be heated in the liquid of choice and they dissolve. Usually 1 tablespoon of agar flakes per 1 cup of liquid is needed to create a gel state, or "kanten," as it is called. Agar-agar provides necessary bulk for regulating the intestines.

- *Arame.* Arame is a tasty black vegetable that comes in thin slivers or strands. It has a sweet, exotic flavor that is wonderful when cooked with other vegetables, such as carrots or onions. Prepare arame by soaking it to remove any sand or dirt. Once it is rehydrated, lift it out of the remaining water, and add a small amount of the arame to a stir-fry recipe, soup, stew, or pressed salad. Arame can also be cooked alone, or with carrots, onions, or lemon juice, for 30 minutes. Arame is rich in vitamins A and B, carbohydrates, calcium, many other minerals, and trace elements.

- *Dulse.* High in iron and iodine, dulse has a tangy, salty flavor that complements vegetables, grains, stews, and fruit dishes. Dry roasted, it becomes a crunchy, savory condiment. Prepare dulse by wiping it with a damp towel to remove any excess salt and sand. Spread it on a cooking sheet and place it in a 250°F oven for 10 minutes. Dulse is rich in protein; vitamins A, C, E, and B; iodine; other minerals; and trace elements.

- *Hijiki.* With a robust flavor and bold appearance, hijiki is a string-like vegetable that is eaten as a side dish. Leftover hijiki is excellent in salads. Prepare hijiki by soaking a small amount in water for about 10 minutes, or until it is rehydrated and soft. Lift it out of the water, rather than pouring the water off, to allow any residues to settle to the bottom of the bowl. Then boil it alone or with carrots, onions, daikon radish, or beans for 1 to 1½ hours. Hijiki is abundant in nutrients, especially protein, the B vitamins, vitamin A, calcium, phosphorous, iron, and many trace elements. It is traditionally used to strengthen the bones and to revitalize the skin and hair. It also helps build strong intestines.

- *Irish moss.* This sea vegetable is used as a thickening agent for soups and stews. It is rich in vitamins A and B_1, iron, sodium, calcium, and other elements.

- *Kombu.* This stalk-like sea vegetable adds sweetness and hardiness to dishes. Use it in soups or cook it as a vegetable with carrots, onions, rutabagas, turnips, or daikon radish. When added to vegetables, beans, or grains, it greatly enhances their flavor, as well as softening them and increasing their digestibility. In addition, its nutrients leach during cooking and infuse the other foods. Prepare kombu by rinsing it in water. It can be used in whole form or chopped into small pieces. When soaked or added to soup, it will expand. When used in longer-cooked dishes, it usually will dissolve.

- *Nori and sushi nori.* Nori is the easiest sea vegetable to use and the one that newcomers to sea vegetables enjoy instantly. Nori, which comes in sheets, is commonly eaten in Japanese restaurants and used to wrap sushi. It can be roasted over an open flame in less than a minute and crumpled up to make a condiment. It is loaded with nutrients, including vitamins A, B, C, and D, calcium, phosphorous, iron, and trace elements.

- *Sea palm.* Native to California, sea palm consists of luscious strands of seaweed with a sweet flavor. It can be used raw, cut into strips and added to salads. It can be boiled, both alone and with other vegetables. When added to soups and stews, it has a softening effect similar to that of kombu. It can also be roasted and ground with sunflower seeds for a delicious crunchy condiment.

- *Wakame.* Wonderful in miso and other soups and stews, wakame enriches the flavor of other vegetables, such as carrots and onions. It also functions as a gentle sweetener. Wakame is leafy and slippery in texture. It expands when soaked, so one "square" is usually sufficient. It is best when soaked, chopped, and added to soups. When boiled, it is fully cooked in 20 minutes. Loaded with nutrients, wakame is high in calcium, thiamine, niacin, and vitamin B_{12}. It is traditionally used in Oriental medicine to purify the blood and strengthen the skin, hair, and intestines.

Beans and Bean Products

Beans are seeds that grow inside pods. They are removed from the pods and dried. They are higher in protein and fat and lower in complex carbohydrates than grains. The vegetable proteins in beans are much easier to digest than animal proteins. Beans should make up between 10 and 15 percent of your daily food intake.

If you suffer from IBD, introduce beans slowly into your diet. Soak the beans overnight in hot water to make them softer and far more digestible. Cook them according to their dryness. The drier the bean, the longer it needs to be soaked and cooked.

As a general rule, soak hard (dry) beans for 6 to 8 hours and cook them for 4 hours. Hard beans include chickpeas and black, white, and yellow soybeans. Soak medium beans for 2 to 4 hours and cook them for 2 hours. Medium beans include azuke, pinto, kidney, navy, black turtle, and lima beans. Soak soft beans as necessary and cook them for 1 hour. Soft beans include green and red lentils, mung beans, and split peas. To boil beans, use 4 cups of water for every 1 cup of beans.

Beans can also be pressure-cooked. When pressure-cooking beans, use 2 cups of water for every 1 cup of beans. Soak hard beans for 2 hours and cook them for 1½ to 2 hours. Soak medium beans for 1 hour and cook them for 1 hour. Soak soft beans for 30 minutes and cook them for 45 minutes.

Cook beans with extra liquid so they will be easier to mash and strain. Mashing and straining removes the outer skin, which is usually what irritates the intestines of sensitive people. Add a small strip of kombu seaweed to the beans at the start of cooking. The kombu will help to tenderize the beans and its minerals will increase their digestibility.

When adding beans to your diet, begin with the varieties that contain the least fat, such as azuki beans, lentils, and chickpeas. Add tamari, shoyu, or salt at the end of cooking to ensure that the beans become soft.

Also good for people with IBD are the bean products tofu and tempeh. Tofu and tempeh are nourishing alternatives to meat, poultry, and dairy products. Tofu readily absorbs the flavors and aromas of the food with which it is cooked and therefore is quite versatile. It is an easier protein to digest due to the soybeans having been thoroughly cooked and it is one of my favorites.

Tempeh is a whole fermented soy food. Made from cooked soybeans that are skinned and held together as a beany mash, it has the texture of a burger. Tempeh can be boiled in soups, steamed, or fried. It should be steamed for 20 minutes before being cooked in a recipe. This allows for easier digestion. Tempeh is a natural source of vitamin B_{12} and good for restoring energy and vitality.

Noodles and Pasta

Who doesn't love pasta? There is an endless variety. Look for whole grain or vegetable noodles and avoid those that are highly processed or contain eggs. White pasta creates acid in the intestines. Being Spanish, I was thrilled to be able to substitute better quality pasta. There is nothing more satisfying and nourishing than a tasty pasta dish. Even when inflamed, my intestines did well with the better quality noodles.

Among the noodles that can be consumed on a regular basis are:

- *Soba.* A rich and hearty buckwheat noodle. It is delicious in soups or boiled and then sautéed with vegetables.
- *Udon.* A hearty whole wheat noodle. It can be used in soups, cooked with vegetables, or boiled and then fried with vegetables.
- *Somen.* A fine brown rice noodle very similar to angel hair pasta. Boil it, with or without vegetables.

Seitan

Often referred to as wheat meat, seitan is the gluten of whole wheat thoroughly kneaded and marinated in tamari or shoyu. For people with IBD, it should be avoided until intestinal health has improved significantly.

Seitan is easier to digest than bread and is an ideal substitute for animal food due to its meaty texture. High in protein, it is very filling and gives strength and vitality. Homemade seitan is far superior in taste and texture to store-bought seitan. Seitan should be eaten only occasionally at first, due to its gluten content.

Breads

Breads provide rapidly absorbed carbohydrates, which elevate the insulin and blood glucose levels, and add weight. All of these factors slow or prevent intestinal healing, especially in people with inflammatory conditions. Until your intestinal health is improved, avoid bread or eat as little as possible. If you eat it at all, steam it first for 1 to 2 minutes. Chew bread until it turns into a liquid in your mouth before swallowing.

Fish

White fish and salmon are the only recommended animal foods. You can have fish in portions of up to 4 ounces two to three times per week. If you need more protein for strength, have fish more often. The best time of the day to eat fish is at midday, when the body can best break it down and digest it.

Fish provides protein, energy, and the omega-3 fatty acids, which promote healing and are essential for healthy digestion. Steaming, poaching, boiling, and pan-frying are all acceptable cooking methods for people with IBD.

If you wish to continue eating chicken or beef, make sure it is free range and as fresh as possible. Eat these foods only in small portions. Marinate meats thoroughly in soy sauce and ginger, and cook them stew style with lots of root vegetables. Eat animal protein with grated daikon radish as a side dish. It will help your intestines break down the fat and protein for easier digestibility. Never eat animal food away from home—you put your life at risk because you don't know what you're getting!

Fruit

Fruit is a natural detoxifier. It cools and relaxes the organs, especially the liver. Fruit is high in enzymes and vitamins, especially vitamin C. It is also rich in sugar. Fruits that grow in temperate climates contain 10 to 12 percent sugar. Tropical and citrus fruits contain 20 to 60 percent sugar. The sugar in fruit creates an overly acidic intestinal condition. It's best to cook the fruit and to add a pinch of salt to help neutralize the acid.

The biggest danger associated with fruit is its high chemical content, with strawberries among the most adulterated of fruits. Many times it's not the seeds that irritate the intestines, but the fungicide methylbromaline. This chemical is so toxic that by law it can only be released underground to the roots of the plants. Take care to eat only seasonal organic fresh fruit and then just occasionally.

Smaller fruits contain more nutrients and less sugar than large fruits. Eat fruit as a snack between meals. Fruit is digested more quickly than other foods, so it's best to eat it alone. Otherwise, the other food will ferment it in your stomach. Do not eat fruit at all until your IBD symptoms have diminished. Introduce dry cooked fruit first and then add fresh cooked fruit as your digestion allows. Add kuzu to the fruit to balance out the sugar and acid content.

Ground fruits that can be enjoyed by people with settled IBD include:

Blackberries	Raisins
Blueberries	Raspberries
Cantaloupes	Strawberries
Honeydew melons	Watermelons

Tree fruits that can be enjoyed by people with settled IBD include:

Apples	Peaches
Apricots	Pears
Cherries	Plums
Grapes	Tangerines

Fruits that should be avoided by people with IBD due to their high sugar and acid content include:

Bananas   Mangos
Coconuts   Papayas
Dates   Pineapples
Figs

Nuts

A nut is a fruit consisting of an oily kernel in a hard shell. Nuts energize. They help build body mass and strength. Nuts are high in protein and vitamin E. They are best used sparingly—if at all—by people with a compromised liver or digestive system, a yeast problem, or a weight problem. To improve the digestibility of nuts, roast them before use and only use them in cooking at first.

Nuts that can be enjoyed by people with settled IBD include:

Almonds   Pecans
Chestnuts   Walnuts
Hazelnuts

Seeds

A seed is like the "egg" of a plant. It contains an embryo and when fertilized will produce a new plant. Seeds are wonderful condiments on grains. Roasting helps to make them more digestible. Limit the amount of seeds you eat to less than half a cup three times a week, depending on their effects on your intestinal condition. Because seeds are small and hard, they often irritate sensitive stomach and intestinal linings.

Seeds that can be enjoyed by people with IBD include:

- *Pumpkin seeds.* Also known as *pepita,* pumpkin seeds originated in South and Central America. Rich in zinc, the omega-3 fatty acids, and vitamin E, they support the male sexual organs, especially the prostate gland. They are higher in protein than any other seed or nut and are also excellent sources of iron, phosphorus, vitamin A, calcium, and some of the B vitamins. Pumpkin seeds energize the spleen, pancreas, liver, and colon. Eaten raw, they help expel pinworms and other intestinal parasites.

- *Sesame seeds.* The sesame is the oldest known plant grown for its seeds. When buying sesame seeds, look for unhulled seeds. Hulled seeds lose their calcium content, as well as their fiber, potassium and iron contents.

  Sesame seeds derive 35 percent of their calories from protein. They have a high vitamin-E content, which helps resist oxidation. They contain as much iron as liver and abundant quantities of the amino acids methionime and tryptophan. They also contain oxalix acid, so should be soaked overnight and then roasted, which removes this unwanted substance. Sesame seeds are used to build a deficient liver and kidneys.

- *Sunflower seeds.* Harvested from the beautiful sunflower, sunflower seeds are considered an energy tonic. They promote healthy bowel elimination and are traditionally used to treat constipation. They contain more protein ounce for ounce than beef. Sunflower seeds are a good source of calcium, phosphorus, and iron, as well as vitamins A, D, and E and several of the B vitamins.

Oils

Oils enhance the flavor of foods and provide balance to meals. They also help to satisfy the appetite. Oil is liquid fat, which means you must be prudent when using it. Use only cold-pressed, unrefined vegetable oils. Vegetable oils contain vitamins A and E. Flaxseed oil and canola oil also contain the omega-3 fatty acids, which are anticancer and immune enhancing. The other vegetable oils contain the omega-6 fatty acids, which are immune depressing.

Most vegetable oils—such as sesame, corn, and safflower oils—are composed primarily of polyunsaturated fats, with small amounts of mono- and saturated fats. Polyunsaturated fats lower the blood cholesterol levels. Saturated fats raise blood cholesterol. Monounsaturated fat has little or no effect on the overall cholesterol level, but may slightly raise the good cholesterol, known as high-density lipoproteins, or HDL. Keep in mind that excessive use of polyunsaturated oils can weaken the immune system and raise your risk of cancer.

How much oil is too much? When you are first recovering from an IBD, use oils sparingly, only twice a week. Instead, water-sauté, boil, or steam your vegetables. As your health improves, you can increase your use of oils. I recommend that when sautéing with oil, only brush the pan lightly with the oil; once the food is cooking then add water, for an oil-and-water sauté. Sauté vegetables only two or three times a week. If you use oil as a condiment, use only about a half-teaspoon on a single serving of vegetables or salad. Again, do this only once or twice a week.

Choose only the highest-quality oils that are cold pressed, virgin, and have no artificial ingredients. Many commercial oils are degummed (washed in a highly caustic solution, such as lye), bleached, and deiodonized. Their natural taste, aroma, and nutrients are lost. They are also flavorless and colorless.

Many margarines and other oil-based foods contain hydrogenated fats. Hydrogenation is a process in which hydrogen atoms are stuffed into the fat molecule, making the fat more saturated and the product thicker and more like butter. This type of oil is immune-depressing, carcinogenic, and a major promoter of heart disease. Avoid hydrogenated oils entirely.

The symptoms of poor oil digestion include bloating, belching, flatulence, and thirst. To help your body better digest oil, grate a little daikon radish, ginger root, or umeboshi plum and eat it with your oil-containing meal.

Among the oils are the following:

- *Canola oil.* Made from the rape plant, canola oil is genetically engineered and originally was used primarily as cattle feed. In 1980 a Canadian oil manufacturer saw the market potential and changed the oil's name from "rapeseed oil" to "canola oil." Canola oil is highly refined and can be toxic, especially for people who have weak digestion and are sensitive to oils and fats.

- *Corn oil.* Unrefined corn oil has a rich buttery flavor and smooth consistency. The darker oil comes from the corn kernel, while the lighter oil comes from the germ. Corn oil is great for baking. However, do not use it for deep-frying because it foams easily.
- *Flax oil.* A great source of the omega-3 fatty acids, flax oil is a drying oil and should not be heated. It is best eaten raw over salads, in dressings, or drizzled over steamed vegetables. Flax oil helps support thyroid, adrenal, and hormone activity. It strengthens the immune system and plays a critical role in healthy brain function.
- *Olive oil.* Derived from a fruit, olive oil is considered more yin in nature than most oils. It is heavier and fattier than the other oils. Olive oil is high in vitamin E and monounsaturated fat, which lowers the bad cholesterol (low-density lipoprotein, or LDL). It helps support liver and gallbladder function. Olive oil is best used only occasionally, on salad or for stir frying. During the healing process, do not use olive oil at all.
- *Safflower oil.* A very mild oil, safflower oil tends to spoil easily. However, it is very stable when heated and is great for deep-fried dishes such as tempura. Safflower oil contains predominantly omega-6 fatty acids. When purchasing safflower oil, look for oleic-rich safflower oil.
- *Sesame oil.* Unrefined sesame oil is ideal for every-day cooking and baking. It is high in vitamin E, and is easier to digest. It is delicious when used for sautéing, in sauces, and in spreads. Dark sesame oil has a robust taste; a little goes a long way. Lighter-colored sesame oil is milder in taste. Sesame oil is highly stable and resistant to spoiling. However, it should still be refrigerated or stored in a cool, dark place.

As long as you are careful not to overdo your oil consumption, you should find that good-quality vegetable oils are a wonderful addition to your cooking. They will enrich the flavor and the experience of your food, making it more fulfilling and satisfying.

* * *

At first, many people view the macrobiotic diet as a temporary detour from the standard American diet. They see a regimen based on grains and vegetables as a source of deprivation, a medicinal diet, meant only to help them overcome some major illness. Certainly that was how I approached the diet when I began. But as I got to know the foods better, and my cooking improved, I began to enjoy this way of eating more and more. Now, I choose to eat a macrobiotic diet not because I have to for my health, but because the foods are delicious to me. The diet provides me with the same satisfaction and enjoyment as my old American diet, and even more, because the macrobiotic foods leave me feeling strong, healthy, and alive.

One of the keys to making this transition—that is, from considering the diet a temporary approach to your normal way of life—is to learn how to prepare the foods. My advice is to take some cooking classes from an experienced macrobiotic cooking teacher. Also, give your palate time to adjust to the new flavors. With a little time and a growing expertise, you will find this diet to be a most delicious and satisfying way of eating. Meanwhile, your health will grow stronger, your symptoms will abate, and eventually you will find yourself free to enjoy and fully participate in your life.

12

Healing Recipes

In this chapter, you will find almost 40 healing macrobiotic recipes, which can form the basis for a whole new way of life. These recipes are meant to serve as an introduction to macrobiotic cooking. For more recipes, see the many wonderful macrobiotic cookbooks that provide more advanced recipes and a wider array of choices.

The recipes that follow will get you going on your macrobiotic diet. As your cooking skills improve and your palate adapts, you will find yourself enjoying these foods more and more. You will also witness a dramatic transformation in your health.

Before you begin your macrobiotic diet, please take note of just two recommendations. First, instead of three large meals per day, eat four to six small, or mini, meals. These small meals will place less stress on your digestion, while promoting healing.

Second, experiment to find the water content and food consistency that are best for your condition. When necessary, run your grains, vegetables, and beans through a blender or food mill. A food mill in particular will remove the excess fiber from food and make it much gentler on your digestion. Do this for as long as necessary, gradually including more and more whole, unprocessed grains, vegetables, and beans that have not been milled. You must retrain your body, especially your digestive tract, to accept whole, unprocessed foods. To make the transition easier, use extra water in your cooking to make your grains, beans, and vegetables softer and easier to digest. Use this extra water especially when you first begin this diet.

Be patient, and enjoy your discovery of macrobiotic cooking. And remember: Chew well!

Breakfast Dishes

Creamed Grain

5 cups water
½ cup presoaked grain (rice, whole oats, millet, or sweet brown rice)
Pinch sea salt
Dried fruit to taste (optional)

Crushed presoaked pumpkin seeds to taste (optional)
Rice syrup or barley malt to taste (optional)
¼ teaspoon flax oil (optional)
Amazake to taste (optional)

In a large saucepan, combine the water, grain, and salt. Bring to a boil over a high flame, then reduce the flame, cover the saucepan, and simmer for 1 hour or until most of the water has been absorbed. If your condition allows, add dried fruit and/or pumpkin seeds during the last few minutes of cooking and for sweetness, add rice syrup or barley malt. For a creamy texture, add flax oil. For a creamy texture and sweetness, add amazake. These may be added at the end.

YIELD: 1 SERVING

Cooked Greens

¼ cup water
1 cup greens (such as broccoli, cabbage, or bok choy)
Sea salt to taste (optional)

Umeboshi vinegar to taste (optional)
Shoyu to taste (optional)

In a medium-sized saucepan, bring the water to a boil over a high flame. Add the greens, reduce the flame, and cover the sauce-pan. Cook for 10 minutes or until the vegetable is soft enough for your digestive system to break down. If desired, season with salt, umeboshi vinegar, or shoyu.

YIELD: 1 SERVING

French Crêpes

2 cups whole wheat pastry flour   ¼ teaspoon sea salt
2 cups water   Dark sesame oil

In a medium-sized bowl, combine the flour, water, and salt; mix with a hand mixer or in a blender to make a lighter batter, adding the oil as necessary. Lightly oil a small skillet or griddle and preheat. Ladle about ⅔ cup of the batter into the heated skil-let and smooth it out with the back of a spoon to form a circular shape. The crêpe should be very thin. Cook the crêpe for 5 min-utes or until done; be careful not to burn it. Carefully peel the crêpe from the skillet and place on a plate. Fill with your favorite filling (for example, scrambled tofu, fruit with kuzu, or stir-fried vegetables), roll up, and fasten with a toothpick. These crêpes are a light way to consume flour. Most digestive systems can han-dle them. For even better crêpes, prepare the batter the night before.

YIELD: 6 SERVINGS

Miso Soup

2 cups water
1/4 cup chopped leek
1/4 cup thinly sliced daikon
1-inch piece dry wakame,
    presoaked and chopped

1/2 teaspoon nonpasteurized
    paste

In a medium-sized saucepan, bring the water to a boil over a high flame. Add the leek, daikon, and wakame, then reduce the flame, cover the saucepan, and gently boil for 10 minutes. Pour about 1/2 cup of the cooking water into a small bowl, add the miso, and stir until dissolved. Pour the miso mixture into the saucepan and turn off the flame; do not boil the miso or the beneficial bacteria will be killed. If the vegetables are too hard on your digestion, remove them and just drink the broth.

YIELD: **2** SERVINGS

Noodles and Broth

(From *Aveline Kushi's Complete Guide to Macrobiotic Cooking*)

10–12 cups water
8-ounce package soba or udon
    noodles
2 dried shiitake mushrooms
    without stems, presoaked and
    sliced

2–3-inch-piece kombu
1/4 package tofu, cubed
    (optional)
3 tablespoons tamari
Chopped scallion or chives
    for garnish

In a large saucepan, bring 6–8 cups water to a boil over a high flame. Add the noodles, lower the flame, and cook for about 10 minutes or until the noodles are done. Meanwhile, in a separate saucepan, combine 4 cups water, mushrooms, and kombu. Bring to a boil over a high flame, then lower the flame and simmer for 5 minutes. Add the tofu and tamari, and simmer for 5 more minutes or until the tofu floats to the top. To serve, divide the noodles between 2 bowls and pour in the broth. Garnish with the scallions or chives. The tofu makes this dish very strengthening. For an even more strengthening dish, replace the tofu with bonito fish flakes.

YIELD: 2 SERVINGS

Oatmeal

1½ cups water
½ cup rolled oats
Pinch sea salt
Amazake, rice syrup, barley malt,
   or flax oil to taste (optional)

Chopped dried or fresh fruit
   to taste (optional)

In a medium-sized saucepan, bring the water to a boil over a high flame. Stir in the oats and salt, then reduce the flame, cover the saucepan, and gently boil for 15–20 minutes or until creamy. If desired, flavor with amazake, rice syrup, barley malt, or flax oil before covering the saucepan, and/or add fruit during the last few minutes of cooking.

YIELD: 2 SERVINGS

Overnight Whole Oats

1½ cups water
¼ cup presoaked whole oats or
   oat groats
Pinch sea salt
Dried fruit to taste (optional)
Crushed preroasted pumpkin
   seeds to taste (optional)

Rice syrup or barley malt to
   taste (optional)
¼ teaspoon flax oil (optional)
Amazake to taste (optional)

The night before, combine the water, oats, and salt in a medium saucepan. Bring to a boil over a high flame, then reduce the flame, cover the saucepan, and simmer gently for 45 minutes. Turn the flame off and let the covered saucepan sit overnight. The oatmeal should be done in the morning. If it's not, cook for an extra 15 minutes or until done. If your condition allows, add dried fruit during the last few minutes of cooking and garnish with roasted pumpkin seeds. For sweetness, add rice syrup or barley malt during the last few minutes. For a creamy texture, add flax oil. For a creamy texture and sweetness, add amazake. These may be added at the end.

YIELD: **2** SERVINGS

Puffed Mochi

¼ mochi square
Apple butter, rice syrup, or
*   barley malt to taste*

Soy sauce to taste (optional)
Crushed pumpkin seeds to
*   taste (optional)*

Brush a skillet with oil and heat over a low flame. Place the mochi in the skillet, cover, and cook for 15 minutes. Do not remove the lid until the mochi is puffy or the mochi will go flat. Slide the mochi onto a plate and top with apple butter, rice syrup, or barley malt. If desired, add soy sauce and/or pumpkin seeds. Puffed mochi is good for muscle tone.

YIELD: **1** SERVING

Scrambled Tofu

¼ teaspoon sesame oil
½ cup chopped scallions or leeks

1 package firm tofu, mashed
Shoyu to taste

Brush a skillet with the oil and heat over a medium-low flame. Add the scallions or leaks, and sauté for 2–3 minutes. Add the tofu and stir to mix. Add the shoyu, cover, and cook for 5 minutes. Check consistency; if too dry, add more shoyu or water. Stir and cook for another 5 minutes. This is a delicious substitute for scrambled eggs. Serve it with grits and miso soup.

YIELD: **4** SERVINGS

Sesame Waffles

(From *Self-Healing Cookbook* by Kristina Turner)

1½ cups oat flakes
1½ cups fine cornmeal
¼ cup toasted sesame seeds
2 cups water

¼ cup cooked millet
1 tablespoon sesame oil
¼ teaspoon sea salt
Apple Syrup (see recipe below)

In a skillet, lightly roast the oat flakes and cornmeal by stirring over a medium flame until nutty-smelling; do not brown. Set aside. In a blender, grind the sesame seeds to a fine powder. Add the roasted oat flakes and cornmeal along with the water, millet, oil, and salt, and blend until smooth. Add more water if the batter is too dry. Oil a waffle iron and preheat. Ladle the batter into the heated waffle iron and cook until golden brown. Slide onto a plate and top with Apple Syrup.

YIELD: 6 SERVINGS

Apple Syrup

(From *Self-Healing Cookbook* by Kristina Turner)

1 cup apple juice
1 heaping tablespoon kuzu
⅓ cup water

2–4 tablespoons rice syrup
Fresh peaches or berries
(optional)

In a small saucepan, heat the apple juice over a low flame. In a small bowl, dissolve the kuzu in the cold water; add gradually to the hot juice, stirring until smooth. Stir in the rice syrup. If the syrup is too thick, add more apple juice.

YIELD: 1¾ CUPS

Steamed Sourdough Bread

1 slice good-quality sourdough   Flax oil or apple butter
   bread (or another yeast-free
   bread such as spelt bread)

Steam the bread slice for 3 minutes using your favorite method. Serve it topped with flax oil or apple butter.

YIELD: 1 SERVING

A Sample Balanced Breakfast

Tea
Hot whole grain porridge
Vegetable (preferably green)
Miso soup

Using this basic menu, you can prepare a delicious and satisfying first meal of the day. Remember that variety is just as important as balance.

Lunch Dishes

Baked Squash

1 small- or medium-sized hard   Shoyu to taste
   winter squash (butternut,   Chopped scallions for garnish
   kabocha, or hokadio)   1 tablespoon grated mochi
Water   (optional)
Flax oil to taste

Preheat the oven to 350°F. Wash the squash, cut it into halves or quarters depending on its size, and remove the seeds. Fill a large baking pan with 1½ inches of water and arrange the squash pieces facedown. Place in the oven and bake for 30–40 minutes or until done. Remove the baking pan from the oven and turn the squash pieces faceup. Scoop the squash meat into a large bowl, add the flax oil and shoyu, and mix. Stuff the squash shells with the meat mixture, arrange on a serving platter, and garnish with the scallions. For a heartier taste, sprinkle with the grated mochi, which will melt and provide a cheesy consistency. This dish is very tasty and soothing to the intestines, and should be eaten often.

YIELD: **3** SERVINGS

Barley Vegetable Soup

2 quarts + 1 cup water
2-inch-piece kombu, rinsed
½ cup pearl barley, rinsed
1 small onion, chopped
1 small parsnip, chopped

1 small carrot, chopped
½ leek, chopped
¼ teaspoon sea salt
½ level teaspoon miso

In a large saucepan, bring 2 quarts water and kombu to a boil over a high flame. Add the barley and bring to a boil again. Add the onion, parsnip, and carrot, and return to a boil. Cover, reduce the flame, and simmer for 25 minutes or until the barley is soft. Add the leek and the salt, and cook for 5 more minutes. In a small bowl, dissolve the miso in 1 cup water; add to the soup, and simmer for 3 minutes. To increase digestibility of this dish, process the soup in a blender.

YIELD: **4** SERVINGS

Black Bean Burritos

4 corn tortillas
Black beans, cooked and creamed
Chopped scallions
Sprouts

Chopped sautéed cabbage
Leftover rice
Sauerkraut

Steam the tortillas until soft. Fill with the remaining ingredients and roll up.

YIELD: 4 SERVINGS

Boiled Cauliflower and Broccoli with Ginger Sauce

Water
1 cup cauliflower florets
1 cup broccoli florets
1 teaspoon shoyu

½ teaspoon grated fresh ginger
1 tablespoon fresh lemon juice
½ cup water

Put 2 inches of water in a medium-sized saucepan and bring to a boil over a high flame. Add the cauliflower and cook until soft; do not overcook. Remove the cauliflower, place in a medium-sized bowl, and set aside. Cook the broccoli and add to the bowl with the cauliflower. In a small bowl, combine the remaining ingredients; pour over the vegetables and toss.

YIELD: 2 SERVINGS

Boiled Millet

1 cup millet
Sesame oil
Chopped onions or other
   vegetables to taste

2½ cups boiling water
Pinch sea salt

Wash the millet and set aside. Brush a large skillet with sesame oil and heat over a high flame. Add the onions and then the millet, and cook, stirring often, until the millet is lightly roasted and its aroma is released. Add the boiling water and salt, and return to a boil. Cover, reduce the flame, and simmer for 35 minutes. This dish is a soft and gentle way to consume vegetables.

YIELD: 4 SERVINGS

Creamed Corn

8 cups + ¼ cup water
4 ears corn, kernels removed
Pinch sea salt

Flax oil to taste
¼ teaspoon kuzu

In a large saucepan, bring 8 cups of water to a boil over a high flame. Add the corn kernels and salt, and cook for 15 minutes. Remove from the flame and drain, reserving the water. Place the mixture in a blender and process until creamy, adding the oil and reserved cooking water as necessary. Pour the mixture back into the saucepan and set aside. In a small bowl, dissolve the kuzu in ¼ cup cold water; add slowly to the creamed corn. Turn on the flame again and cook, stirring, until the kuzu is clear and well mixed. For an even creamier texture, strain the creamed corn before adding the kuzu.

YIELD: 2 SERVINGS

Cucumber Wakame Salad

1½ cups water
1 cup presoaked wakame
2 cups sliced cucumber

Shoyu to taste
Brown rice vinegar to taste
Grated fresh ginger to taste

In a medium-sized saucepan, bring the water to a boil over a high flame. Add the wakame and boil for 2 minutes; drain, cool slightly, and chop. In a large bowl, combine the wakame and cucumber slices. Add the shoyu, brown rice vinegar, and ginger, and toss. Let sit for 5 minutes to allow the cucumber slices to pickle.

YIELD: 2 SERVINGS

Kimpira (Sautéed and Simmered Vegetables)

Sesame oil
1 cup burdock, washed and cut
   into matchsticks
1 cup carrots, washed and cut
   into matchsticks

Pinch sea salt
Water
Shoyu
Fresh ginger juice

Lightly brush a large skillet with sesame oil and heat over a high flame. Add the burdock, then the carrots, and finally the salt, and sauté for 3 minutes. Add just enough water to cover the bottom of the skillet. Add several drops of the shoyu, cover the skillet, and cook for 10 minutes or until the water has almost evaporated. Add a few drops of the ginger juice, stir, and remove from the flame. This dish should be eaten often because it promotes strength and vitality. For an even more strengthening dish, add presoaked arame or hijiki right after the carrots.

YIELD: 4 SERVINGS

Koi-Kuku (Fish Soup)

(From *Aveline Kushi's Complete Guide to Macrobiotic Cooking*.)

1 fresh trout, cleaned
Burdock root
½ cup used bancha twigs,
  wrapped in cheesecloth
Bancha tea

Water
Miso
1 tablespoon grated fresh
  ginger

Remove the eyes from the trout and cut the meat into 1- to 2-inch-thick slices. Cut an equal amount of burdock root into thin matchsticks. Place the fish slices and burdock pieces in a pressure cooker, top with the bancha twigs, and add enough of the bancha tea and water, in equal amounts, to cover the fish. Pressure-cook for 1 hour, then let the pressure down and add ½–1 teaspoon miso per cup of soup. Add the ginger and simmer for 5 minutes; do not boil. This soup is excellent for restoring strength and vitality. The bancha twigs help to soften the fish bones during cooking and make them more digestible. Eat the soup in small amounts; freeze the leftover.

YIELD: **2** QUARTS

Lentils

1-inch-piece kombu, rinsed
½ cup diced burdock
½ cup diced carrots
¼ cup diced celery
1 cup dry lentils, rinsed

2½ cups water
1½ teaspoons tamari or shoyu
Chopped parsley or scallions for
  garnish

Place the kombu in the bottom of a large saucepan. On top of the kombu, layer the diced burdock, carrots, and celery. Layer the lentils on top of the vegetables and add the water to cover. Bring the mixture to a boil over a high flame, then reduce the flame to medium-low, cover the saucepan, and simmer for 45 minutes. Season with the tamari and simmer for 5 more minutes or until the lentils are soft. To serve, garnish with the parsley or scallions. Lentils are gentle on the digestion. This dish is also a good way to incorporate root vegetables into the diet, since they are cooked for a substantial period of time, increasing their digestibility.

YIELD: 3 SERVINGS

Millet Croquettes

1 cup leftover cooked millet
Grated carrot to taste
Grated onion to taste
Cornmeal to taste

Dark sesame oil
Tofu mayonnaise or mustard
*   as garnish*

In a bowl, mix the millet, carrot, and onion together. Add just enough cornmeal so the millet mixture can be formed into a patty. Pour enough oil into a skillet to cover the bottom and heat over a medium flame. Add the patty and cook until browned. Flip the patty and brown the other side. Serve with the tofu mayonnaise or mustard.

YIELD: 1 SERVING

Noodle Salad with Lemon Vinaigrette

Water
8-ounce package buckwheat or
*   brown rice noodles*
½ cup daikon, cut into
*   matchsticks*
½ cup carrot, cut into
*   matchsticks*

1 bunch watercress
1 tablespoon dried arame
Pinch sea salt
Lemon Vinaigrette to taste
*   (see recipe below)*

Fill a large saucepan with water and bring to a boil over a high flame; add the noodles and cook until tender. Meanwhile, in a skillet, sauté or steam the daikon, carrot, watercress, and arame along with the salt until soft. Remove from the flame and set aside to cool until the noodles are done. Drain the noodles and toss in the vegetable mixture and Lemon Vinaigrette.

YIELD: **6** SERVINGS

Lemon Vinaigrette

¼ *cup fresh lemon juice*	*2 teaspoons brown rice vinegar*
¼ *cup water*	*2 teaspoons flax oil*
3 teaspoons shoyu	½ *teaspoon mustard*

In a small bowl, mix all the ingredients until well blended.

YIELD: **2** CUPS

Poached Fish

Shoyu to taste	*Small- to medium-sized piece of orange*
Lemon juice to taste	*roughy or other white-meat fish, rinsed*

In a baking dish, combine the shoyu and lemon juice, and stir. Add the fish and marinate for 20 minutes. The shoyu and lemon juice will draw some of the liquid out of the fish. Brush a large skillet with olive oil and heat over a medium flame. Add the fish and sear for 2 to 3 minutes. Flip the fish and drizzle with the marinade, adding enough to half cover the fish. If more liquid is needed, add more shoyu mixed with water. Cover and cook for 15 minutes or until flaky in the middle.

YIELD: **1** SERVING

A Sample Balanced Lunch

Grain dish
2 vegetable dishes
Protein dish
Soup (optional)
Dessert (optional)
Beverage

Use this basic menu to prepare a delicious and satisfying midday meal. Remember to vary your dishes every day.

Dinner Dishes

Azuki Beans with Squash

1 cup azuki beans
1-inch-piece kombu
2 cups chopped winter squash

Water
Shoyu to taste

Wash the azuki beans and soak them in water with the kombu for at least 5 hours. Remove the kombu, dice it, and sprinkle it on the bottom of a large saucepan. Add the squash and then the azuki beans, cover with water, and bring to a boil over a high flame. Reduce the flame, cover, and cook for about 1 hour or until the beans are soft. Sprinkle with the shoyu and cook for 5 more minutes. Azuki beans help strengthen the kidneys and detoxify the body of drugs.

YIELD: 4 SERVINGS

Boiled Salad

Water
Pinch sea salt
½ cup thinly sliced carrots
½ cup thinly sliced daikon

½ cup finely chopped kale
1 teaspoon umeboshi paste
¼ teaspoon brown rice syrup

Put about 4 inches of water and the salt in a medium-sized saucepan and bring to a boil over a high flame. Add the carrots and cook for 2 minutes or until the color intensifies and the vegetables have softened. Remove the carrots with a slotted spoon and place in a medium-sized bowl. Repeat with the daikon and finally the kale. Ladle out ½ cup of the cooking water and place in a small bowl. Add the umeboshi paste and brown rice syrup, and stir until dissolved. Drizzle over the vegetables and toss before serving.

YIELD: **2** SERVINGS

Hijiki with Tahini Sauce

2 carrots, cut into matchsticks
1 onion, halved and sliced
1 cup presoaked hijiki
3 tablespoons rice syrup

2 tablespoons tahini
2 tablespoons fresh ginger juice
2 tablespoons shoyu
2 teaspoons lemon juice

In a large skillet, water-sauté the carrots, onion, and hijiki for 10 minutes. In a small bowl, combine the rice syrup, tahini, ginger juice, shoyu, and lemon juice. Stir into the skillet, cover, and cook for 5 minutes. Remove from the flame and allow to sit until excess liquid evaporates.

YIELD: **4** SERVINGS

Nishime (Steamed Root Vegetables)

2-inch-piece kombu
½ cup onions, cut into 2-inch chunks
½ cup carrots, cut into 2-inch slices
½ cup parsnip, cut into 2-inch chunks

½ cup winter squash, cut into 2-inch chunks
Water
Shoyu to taste

Place the kombu in the center of the bottom of a large saucepan. Arrange the onions, carrots, parsnip, and squash in separate groups around the kombu. Carefully add 1 inch of water to the saucepan; cover and bring to a boil over a high flame. Reduce the flame and cook for 25 minutes; do not stir and do not lift the lid. If the water evaporates during the cooking, carefully add more water. Drizzle with the shoyu and cook for 5 more minutes or until the vegetables are soft. Remove from the flame and mix. This dish provides stabilizing energy. Root vegetables are strengthening for the intestines, particularly the colon. Therefore, you should eat this dish two to three times a week.

YIELD: 4 SERVINGS

Pressed Salad

1 cup thinly sliced bok choy or Chinese cabbage
¼ cup thinly sliced red radishes

¼ cup thinly sliced celery
½ tablespoon umeboshi vinegar

Place the vegetables in a large bowl and drizzle with the vinegar. Using your hands, mix gently but thoroughly for several minutes; knead as if kneading bread dough. Place a small plate on top of the vegetables in the bowl and put a jug of water or something equally heavy on top of the plate. Let sit for 20 to 30 minutes, then drain off the juice that has been pressed out. Toss the vegetables before serving. This quick pickling method increases the digestibility of raw crunchy vegetables. It also provides digestive enzymes. Therefore, this dish is good to eat two to three times per week.

YIELD: **2** SERVINGS

Pressure-Cooked Brown Rice

2 cups dry rice   ½-inch-piece kombu
4 cups water

In a large bowl, soak the rice in the water for at least 5 hours. Pour the rice and soaking water into a pressure cooker and add the kombu. Pressure-cook for 50 minutes. Pressure-cooking is a strengthening way to eat grains and beans. It increases their digestibility. This dish is good for low energy and weakened conditions.

YIELD: **3** SERVINGS

Variations:

- 80 percent brown rice with 20 percent millet, sweet brown rice, or pearled barley
- 90 percent brown rice with 10 percent azuki beans, black soybeans, or chickpeas

Brown rice is the recommended grain for regular use during the beginning stages of healing. Its energetic properties help strengthen the colon. Use short-grain rice and pressure-cook it. Millet is the second most healing grain and the second most recommended for regular use during healing. It is the most alkalizing grain, and the large intestine needs an alkaline environment to function properly. Pressure-cooking also is the preferred cooking method for millet.

Quinoa with Tempeh

2½ cups + 4 tablespoons water
1 tablespoon shoyu
1 teaspoon fresh ginger juice
1 teaspoon mustard
1 package tempeh, cut into cubes
   and steamed for 15 minutes
1 cup quinoa, cleaned and rinsed

¼ cup chopped red radish
¼ cup chopped celery
¼ cup chopped parsley
¼ cup presoaked arame
Dark sesame oil
1 tablespoon fresh lemon juice
½ teaspoon sea salt

In a medium-sized bowl, combine 2 tablespoons of water, the shoyu, the ginger juice, and the mustard. Add the steamed tempeh and marinate for 15 minutes; drain and set aside. In a medium-sized saucepan, bring 2½ cups of water to a boil over a high flame. Add the quinoa, reduce the flame, and cook for 35 minutes or until done; set aside to cool. In a small skillet, blanche the vegetables one at a time for 1 minute each; set aside to cool. Brush another small skillet with the oil and heat over a high flame. Add the marinated tempeh and pan-fry until browned on all sides. Remove from the skillet and set aside to cool. Fluff the quinoa and transfer to a large bowl. Add the vegetables and tempeh, and stir. In a small bowl, mix together the remaining 2 tablespoons of water, the lemon juice, and the salt. Pour into the quinoa mixture and toss to mix.

YIELD: 4 SERVINGS

Squash and Sweet Potato Bisque

½ winter squash, cut into cubes
2 medium sweet potatoes, cut
   into cubes
Water, as needed

¼ cup teff
½ teaspoon sea salt
½ level teaspoon sweet miso

Place the squash and sweet potatoes in a large saucepan, cover with water, and bring to a boil over a high flame. Reduce the flame to medium-low and cook for 20 minutes or until soft. Mash with a potato masher and add the teff. If the mixture is too thick, add more water. Cook for 10 minutes. Add the salt and cook for 5 more minutes. Transfer the mixture to a blender and process until creamy and smooth. Return to the saucepan and bring back to a boil. In a small bowl, dissolve the miso in 1 cup of water. Add to the saucepan and simmer for 1 minute. This dish is a delicious way to eat vegetables in soup form. Other vegetables that can be turned into similar soups are broccoli and carrots.

YIELD: 4 SERVINGS

Tofu Stir-Fry

Olive oil
½ cup chopped onions
½ cup presoaked hijiki
½ cup chopped broccoli or bok choy
½ cup sliced carrots
½ cup sliced mushrooms
½ cup snap peas
½ package tofu, drained, excess water squeezed out, and cubed
Shoyu or sea salt to taste

Brush a large skillet with olive oil and heat over a high flame. Add the onions and sauté for 2 minutes. Add the hijiki and sauté for 2 more minutes. Add the broccoli, carrots, mushrooms, and snap peas one at a time, sautéing the mixture for 1 to 2 more minutes after each addition. Stir in the tofu, cover, and cook for 10 minutes. Add the shoyu and cook for an additional 10 minutes. Remove from the flame and toss before serving.

YIELD: 2–4 SERVINGS

A Sample Balanced Dinner

Soup (optional)
Whole grain dish
2–3 vegetable dishes (including sea vegetables)
Beans or bean product
Pickles
Dessert (optional)
Beverage

This basic menu can help you prepare a balanced and satisfying dinner. Remember that you can also serve the lunch dishes for dinner, and any of the dinner dishes for lunch.

Dessert Dishes and Beverages

Fresh Juice

Carrots   *Parsley (optional)*
Apple (optional)

Scrub the carrots with a brush, cut off the tops, and cut the carrots into pieces small enough to fit through the hopper of a juice extractor. If using an apple, wash, peel, core, and cut into small chunks. If using parsley, rinse and chop. Prepare a total of 1 cup of carrot pieces, carrot and apple pieces, or carrot pieces and parsley. Juice the vegetables, stir the juice, and pour into a glass. Let sit at room temperature for a few minutes, then drink on an empty stomach. If desired, warm the juice for a sweeter taste and to increase its relaxation effects. Avoid the carrot-apple and carrot-parsley combinations during flare-ups.

YIELD: 1 SERVING

Fruit Kanten

4 cups of your favorite juice   *Dried fruit to taste (optional)*
4 tablespoons kanten flakes
*   (agar-agar)*

In a large saucepan, bring the juice to a boil over a high flame. Add the kanten flakes, reduce the flame, and simmer for 5 minutes or until the kanten flakes have dissolved. Remove from the flame, stir in the fruit, and pour into a pan. Let sit at room temperature or refrigerate until congealed. This dessert has a high mineral content. It is soothing to the intestines and promotes normal bowel activity.

YIELD: **6** SERVINGS

Ginger Handy's Apple Pie

6–8 tart McIntosh apples, grated   *1 teaspoon cinnamon*
¼ cup whole wheat pastry flour   *Pinch sea salt*
¼ cup rice syrup   *Pie Crust (see recipe below)*

Preheat the oven to 350°F. In a large bowl, combine the grated apples, pastry flour, rice syrup, cinnamon, and salt. Pour into the Pie Crust, place in the oven, and bake for 45 minutes.

YIELD: **8** SERVINGS

Pie Crust

Oil
1½ cups whole wheat pastry
   flour
6 tablespoons corn oil

4 tablespoons water
2 tablespoons maple syrup
2 teaspoons arrowroot
¼ teaspoon sea salt

Prepare a 9-inch pie plate by brushing it with oil; set aside. In a large bowl, combine the pastry flour, corn oil, water, maple syrup, arrowroot, and salt; mix with a fork or your hands until well blended. Press the mixture into the prepared pie plate, place in the oven, and bake for 4 minutes. Remove from the oven, add Ginger Handy's Apple Pie or other filling, and bake according to the pie directions.

YIELD: 1 PIE CRUST

Glazed Pears

4 ripe pears, halved
1 cup apple juice
1 tablespoon kuzu dissolved in
   cold water

Pinch sea salt
½ teaspoon grated ginger

Preheat the oven to 350°F. Arrange the pear halves face up in a baking dish. Pour the juice over the pears, cover, and bake until soft. Remove the baking dish from the oven and drain the liquid into a small saucepan; leave the pear halves in the baking dish. Add the kuzu mixture, salt, and ginger to the saucepan and cook over a low flame, stirring constantly, until thick and transparent. Pour over the pears, return the pears to the oven, and bake for 10 more minutes or until glazed.

YIELD: 8 SERVINGS

Peach Custard

3 cups + 2 tablespoons apple juice
1 cup water
6 tablespoons agar-agar flakes
2 cups sliced fresh peaches

2 tablespoons sesame tahini
3 heaping tablespoons kuzu
1 teaspoon vanilla extract

In a large saucepan, bring 3 cups of apple juice, the water, and the agar-agar flakes to a boil over a high flame. Reduce the flame and simmer for 10 minutes. Add the sliced fruit and tahini, and stir to mix. In a small bowl, dissolve the kuzu in 2 tablespoons of unheated apple juice; stir slowly until thickened. Add to the saucepan and stir. Add the vanilla and stir. Pour the mixture into a small bowl and set aside to cool and gel. This dish is a creamy, satisfying dessert that is gentle on the intestines.

YIELD: 4 SERVINGS

Ten-Minute Lemon Pie

Oil
½ cup chopped roasted walnuts
2 cups water
½ cup semolina
8 ounces soft tofu

⅓ cup rice syrup
2 tablespoons lemon juice
1 teaspoon almond extract
Pinch sea salt

Prepare an 8- or 9-inch pie plate by brushing it with oil and lining it with the walnuts; set aside. In a medium-sized saucepan, bring the water to a boil over a high flame. Stir in the semolina, reduce the flame, and cook, covered, for 5 minutes. In a blender, combine the tofu, rice syrup, lemon juice, almond extract, and salt, and process until creamy and smooth. Add to the semolina and stir until creamy. Pour into the prepared pie plate and place in the refrigerator to cool.

YIELD: 8 SERVINGS

Beverages

Always drink beverages at room temperature and avoid drinking them during meals. Helpful beverages to drink are:

- *Spring water.* Drink half your body weight in ounces every day.
- *Bancha kukicha twig tea.* Drink as needed.
- *Fruit juices.* Drink only occasionally. Dilute fruit juices with water and boil them with a pinch of salt to neutralize the acid. Drink them at room temperature.
- *Vegetable juices.* Drink these juices three to four times a week to increase your supply of digestive enzymes. A good vegetable juice is carrot juice.
- *Amazake.* Drink this sweet rice drink warm. It is wonderful as a snack.
- *Roasted barley tea.* Drink this tea often. It is especially enjoyable in the summertime, since it is very cooling to the body.

Avoid drinking cold or iced beverages because they slow the digestion by temporarily halting parastolic movement.

13

Healing Remedies, Supplements, and Lifestyle Practices

Long before the medical and pharmaceutical industries existed as we know them today, natural healers were schooled in the medical traditions of their cultures. Whether Asian, Native American, European, African, or Indian, these healers learned how to use plants, plant extracts, and physical therapies to fight disease and restore health.

For the most part, natural medical therapies were designed to promote the body's own healing mechanisms. It's true that many medicinal plants fight disease directly by providing natural antifungal or antibiotic chemicals. But unlike most of the medicines of today, natural medicine was used essentially to stimulate and restore the body's own healing properties. One of the ways it did this was by restoring the acid-alkaline balance of the blood. Another was by boosting the body's immune defenses. And still another was by promoting the health, vitality, and healing capabilities of the individual organs, such as the small and large intestines.

The natural remedies, supplements, and lifestyle practices discussed in this chapter promote the healing of Crohn's and other IBDs by employing all three of these strategies, to varying degrees. Many of them have been used for thousands of years to promote digestive health and the healing of the intestinal tract. All are substances or practices with which I am extremely familiar and have used myself. All are safe and effective, and most are simple to use and inexpensive. They are all meant to complement, not replace, the care and guidance of a medical doctor.

Healing Remedies

The following traditional healing remedies are meant to be employed in conjunction with a healing diet. They should be used for limited periods of time, for as few as seven days or as long as several months. Traditional healers maintain that healing remedies stimulate the organs to function at a higher rate of efficiency and healthfulness, but that it is better to stop a remedy for a short period of time to allow the organ or system to function at the new level on its own. If you take a remedy for some time, it's a good idea to pause for about a week and see what reaction, if any, your body has to the absence of the herb or therapy. Resume taking the remedy after a few days, if necessary. Be aware that some remedies need to be reduced slowly over time and not stopped abruptly.

Kuzu

Kuzu is the white starch from the root of the wild kudzu plant. It is used to thicken medicinal teas, soups, sauces, and desserts. It is alkalizing and contracting (yang). It strengthens the intestines and intestinal function. Because of its balancing and alkalizing effects, it promotes healing throughout the body. The directions for using kuzu are provided in the descriptions of the individual teas that follow.

Ame-Kuzu Tea

Ame-kuzu tea promotes healing of the stomach and intestines. It relieves cramping, spasms, and constipation. It relaxes the body and mind. To make ame-kuzu tea, dissolve 1 heaping teaspoon of kuzu in 2 teaspoons of water. Add 1 cup of cold water, or ½ cup of water plus ½ cup of apple juice, and bring to a boil over a medium flame, stirring constantly to prevent clumping. If you use just water, stir in 1 teaspoon of rice syrup or barley malt. Continue stirring until the liquid becomes translucent and thickens. Drink the tea hot.

Ume-sho-Kuzu

Ume-sho-kuzu strengthens the intestines and restores energy. It is excellent for controlling diarrhea and bleeding. The looser your diarrhea, the more kuzu you should use. As soon as your symptoms diminish or stop, you can discontinue drinking the ume-sho-kuzu.

Ume-sho-kuzu is especially good for people whose Crohn's or colitis symptoms are active in the morning. If your symptoms follow this pattern, prepare ume-sho-kuzu ahead of time and keep it in a thermos at your bedside. This way, you can drink the beverage before getting out of bed.

To prepare ume-sho-kuzu, dissolve 1 heaping teaspoon of kuzu in 3 tablespoons of water. Pour it into a saucepan along with 1 cup of water and add umeboshi plum that has been chopped into small pieces. Bring the mixture to a boil over a high flame, stirring continuously then reduce the flame to medium-low and simmer until the mixture becomes thickened and translucent. Remove it from the flame, add 3 to 5 drops of shoyu, and gently stir. Drink the beverage hot.

Ume-sho-Kuzu with Ginger

Drink ume-sho-kuzu with ginger when you have diarrhea but no bleeding. To prepare it, follow the recipe for ume-sho-kuzu but add ⅛ teaspoon grated ginger juice before the liquid thickens. Drink the beverage hot. Umesho-kuzu with ginger promotes energy and warmth.

Kuzu Sauce

Kuzu sauce maintains intestinal strength and health. Make it by adding ame-kuzu tea, ume-sho-kuzu, or ume-sho-kuzu with ginger to soup, to the liquid when stir-frying or water sautéing, or to a sauce. See Chapter 12 for some appropriate macrobiotic recipes.

Kukicha Twig Tea

Kukicha twig tea, also known as bancha tea, is a Japanese tea that is alkalizing and soothing, especially to the digestive tract. It has only trace amounts of caffeine, so you can drink it in the evening without fear of it keeping you awake or irritating your intestines. To make the tea, use the twigs, typically referred to as the kukicha, rather than the leaves of the plant. Place 1 tablespoon of twigs in 6 cups of water, bring to a boil, remove from the heat, and let steep for a few minutes. Drink the tea warm or at room temperature. For a stronger taste you can reduce the water.

Umeboshi Plum

Umeboshi plums are pickled plums that have a pungent, sour, salty taste. Highly alkaline, they aid digestion and promote healthy intestinal flora. Add an umeboshi plum to pressure-cooked or boiled grains at the onset of cooking to increase the digestibility of the grain.

Umeboshi Tea

Like ume-sho-kuzu, umeboshi tea is good for people whose Crohn's or colitis symptoms are active in the morning. It helps indigestion, bloating, acid reflux, gassy cramps, and headache. Also like ume-sho-kuzu, umeboshi tea can be prepared ahead of time and kept in a thermos at bedside. To make the tea, pour 1 cup of hot kukicha twig tea over half an umeboshi plum. Steep for a few minutes, then add ¼ teaspoon of shoyu, and drink the tea hot. Umeboshi tea can also be added to pressure-cooked or boiled grains at the onset of cooking to increase their digestibility.

Shoyu

Shoyu is a naturally fermented soy sauce with no artificial ingredients. It is rich in friendly bacteria and digestive enzymes, and aids in the digestions of grains, beans, animal products, and vegetables. Shoyu contains less sodium than tamari, another type of soy sauce, and is suitable for every day use. It is best used in cooking.

Shoyu–Kukicha Twig Tea

Shoyu–kukicha twig tea alkalizes the blood, spleen, and digestion. It relieves fatigue and neutralizes acidity. To prepare shoyu–kukicha twig tea, put 1 teaspoon of shoyu in a mug and add 1 cup of hot kukicha twig tea. Stir the tea and drink it hot.

Ginger Root

Ginger root is an herb with a pungent taste and a firm texture. It can be grated and used in teas or as a garnish for vegetables. Alkalizing and detoxifying, ginger stimulates the liver and cleanses the blood. It warms the body, promotes circulation, dissolves stagnation, and increases the energy flow.

Ginger Tea

Ginger tea is good for nausea and tight cramping pain. To prepare it, grate enough fresh ginger root to make 1 teaspoon of ginger juice. Place the ginger juice in a mug and add 1 cup of hot kukicha twig tea. Drink the tea hot. Note that ginger tea may cause sweating, so should not be used when feverish.

Ginger–Lemon Peel Pickles

Ginger-lemon peel pickles aid digestion, build healthy flora, and stimulate the digestive enzymes. To make ginger-lemon peel pickles, slice the peels from 10 lemons and place in a saucepan. Add ½ cup water and cook, uncovered, for 5 minutes or until the liquid is reduced. Add 1 cup of miso and 1 teaspoon of grated ginger root, mix thoroughly, and sauté for 2–3 minutes. Remove the saucepan from the flame and allow the mixture to cool, then pour the mixture into a glass jar with a tight lid and set it aside to ferment at room temperature for one week. After one week, place the jar in the refrigerator. Discard the excess miso and serve the lemon-peel pickles as a side dish with rice or vegetables. If the lemon peels are too salty, rinse them quickly under water.

Ginger Compress

A hot compress applied to the intestines or other affected area, a ginger compress dissolves stagnation, blockages, and tension, and stimulates blood circulation and energy flow. To make a ginger compress, heat 1 gallon of water over a high flame and bring to boil. Meanwhile, grate enough ginger root to equal the size of a small lemon. When the water is hot, reduce the flame to low, place the grated ginger on a single layer of cheesecloth, tie the cheesecloth with a piece of string or a twist tie, and squeeze the juice from the ginger root into the water. Place the sack of grated ginger in the water and allow the ginger to steep for 5 minutes. Do not boil. Dip a hand towel into the water, leaving its two ends dry so that you can hold the towel without being burned, then wring it out and place it over the affected area. Cover the area with a dry handtowel to deflect the strong heat at first; then you can place the compress directly on the skin. Cover the towel with a dry towel to trap the heat. When the towel cools, repeat the process with the same towel or a new towel. Keep the water hot between dippings, and do not allow the skin to cool between applications. Continue applying compresses for 10 to 15 minutes or until the affected area becomes pink.

Caution: Do not use a ginger compress on the top of the head or for any brain disorder, on the forehead or when temperature is present, on the lower abdomen during pregnancy, for appendicitis pain, or on children younger than five years of age, or on people more than sixty years old.

Shiitake Mushrooms

Shiitake mushrooms are a culinary and medicinal staple in the East. They are available in fresh and dry forms, and are high in minerals, protein, and the B vitamins. Shiitake mushrooms have powerful cholesterol-lowering and anticancer effects. They are effective at reducing fever, dissolving animal fats, relieving tension, and reversing contracted conditions.

Shiitake Tea

Shiitake tea provides all the benefits of shiitake mushrooms. It helps to relieve abdominal cramps and spasms, and reduces fever. To prepare shiitake tea, soak 1 shiitake mushroom in 1 cup of water for 20 minutes. When the mushroom is soft, chop it into very small pieces. Add it to a saucepan containing 1 cup of water that has been brought to a boil and let it simmer for 15 minutes. Strain and pour it into a mug, add a few drops of shoyu, and drink it hot.

Daikon Radish

A daikon radish is a root vegetable also known as a white radish. It is highly versatile and can be eaten either cooked or raw. Traditionally, daikon radish is used to dissolve fats, hardened masses, calcified kidney stones, and blockages in the intestinal tract. It also assists in weight reduction. The best way to prepare daikon radish is to cut it into small slices or matchsticks, and steam or boil it for 5 to 7 minutes. It can be cooked alone or along with other vegetables.

Daikon-Carrot Drink

Daikon-carrot drink is especially helpful in dissolving masses in the intestinal tract of people with Crohn's or colitis. To prepare the drink, place a ½ cup of grated carrot and ½ cup of grated daikon in a saucepan along with 2 cups of water. Bring the mixture to a gentle boil and add ⅓ sheet of nori and ½ umeboshi plum. Simmer the mixture for 3 minutes, then add a few drops of shoyu and remove the saucepan from the flame. Eat the vegetables and drink the broth. For the best results, consume 1 cup of daikon-carrot drink three days in a row, rest for four days, and repeat. Do this for one month. Discontinue consuming the drink if your condition weakens.

Sea Salt

Sea salt is a type of salt that should be used only in cooking. Do not use it in its raw form, since it is prone to crystallizing in the body. Sea salt is essential for healthy blood, lymph, tissue fluids, digestion, and nerve function. It is used in small amounts in cooking to support the kidneys, bladder, heart, and small intestines. Quality is crucial for health when buying sea salt. The brand that I prefer is "Si" salt, found in most natural foods or health food stores.

Salt Pack

A salt pack reduces diarrhea, stomach cramps, and inflammation in the abdomen. To make a salt pack, dry roast 1½ cups of any kind of sea salt (it is best to use a cheap sea salt for this treatment) in a stainless steel skillet until it is very hot. Wrap the hot salt in a thick cotton towel and tie the towel securely with a string. Apply the salt pack to the affected area, changing it when it cools off. Apply a pack three days in a row, rest for two days, and repeat. Sea salt can be used repeatedly. It should be discarded only when it turns gray and can no longer hold heat.

Yarrow

Yarrow is a daisylike plant that grows wild in meadows and alongside roads. It helps stop bleeding and is traditionally used to treat wounds. It also promotes optimal functioning of the circulatory and digestive systems and urinary tract. Yarrow is effective as an infusion for sitz baths and as a compress. It helps reduce the inflammation associated with fistulas and abscesses in the rectal area. It kills harmful bacteria and promotes healing. Yarrow can be used as often as needed. To prepare a yarrow infusion, put 1 cup of dried yarrow in a bowl. Boil 2 quarts of water and pour it over the yarrow. Allow the yarrow to steep for 15 minutes, then strain out the yarrow and allow the liquid to cool. Yarrow needs to be fresh each time it is used.

Healing Supplements

The following supplements are medicinal herbs, in contrast to the remedies just discussed, which are foods. The purpose of taking these supplements is to further assist the healing process. These supplements as a group clean the digestive track of mucus and plaque, which are created by the body to protect itself from acids and toxic compounds, and provide the substances that the body needs for regeneration.

Acidophilous Lactobacillus

Acidophilous lactobacillus, often called just acidophilous, is a prepared formula of friendly bacteria taken orally to replenish the digestion-promoting flora in the intestines. It replenishes the friendly intestinal bacteria killed by medications and antibiotics. A probiotic formula containing bifidobacteria and acidophilous is the best form for colon health. It is essential for healthy immune system function. Use probiotic as needed; most people take it daily. However, do not take acidophilous by itself for more than three months. Acidophilous is an acidic bacteria and, when used indefinitely, may eventually stifle enzymatic function in the small intestine.

Aloe Vera

The aloe vera (*Aloe vera* or *Aloe officinalis*) plant produces an array of medicinal substances in its leaves, which are filled with a thick gel. The gel, which contains 22 amino acids, is used externally to treat wounds, sores, or skin abrasions. It is also converted to a liquid that is taken internally to treat intestinal disorders. The liquid can be purchased in most natural foods and health food stores. It restores digestive function by reducing internal inflammation, penetrating and soothing damaged, infected tissue, and promoting new and healthy cell growth. It also treats mouth ulcers, fistulas, and abscesses. The recommended dosage of aloe vera is 2 to 4 ounces a day when the stools are runny and 4 to 6 ounces a day when the stools are hard. Aloe vera is made in either of two ways. One is the organic whole leaf juice. The other is the organic filet juice. For stronger healing, the organic whole leaf is recommended. For maintenance, the filet is adequate. They also offer aloe in gel form. Don't put yourself through the agony of eating the gel. The gel is the filet juice that has been thickened with carrageenan, a thickener extracted from Irish moss.

Chamomile Tea

Chamomile is derived from the flower of the chamomile plant *(Matricaria chamomillia)*. It is traditionally used to soothe and relax the liver, treat indigestion, and reduce or eliminate bloating. It acts as an anti-inflammatory, relaxes tension, and promotes deep sleep. Chamomile is widely available in tea bags, as a dried herb, and in tinctures. To prepare a cup of tea, steep 1 tablespoon of the dried herb in 1 cup of boiled water for 10 to 20 minutes. Strain out the herb and drink the tea as needed for bloating.

Digestive Enzymes

Digestive enzymes assist digestion by breaking down food for assimilation. They promote optimal function of the small intestine, endocrine system, and thyroid. The three most important digestive enzymes to take are amylase, which helps digest carbohydrates; protease, which helps digest protein; and lipase, which helps digest fats. (For a complete discussion of these digestive enzymes, see Chapter 10.) Take digestive enzymes right before, during, or after every meal. Take higher doses at the beginning of the healing process and taper off to the recommended doses as your condition improves.

Flax Oil

Flax oil is derived from the seeds of the flax plant (*Linum vsitatissmum*). It contains several essential amino acids and is rich in the omega-3 fatty acids. The oil soothes and heals the intestinal tract and serves as a mild laxative. It detoxifies the intestines and helps to maintain their proper function and activity. Since people with IBD have difficulty digesting fats, begin taking flax oil in doses of just ¼ teaspoon every day for three days. Rest for three days, then take ½ teaspoon per day for three days. Rest for another three days and take 1 teaspoon per day for three days.

Continue this way until you reach 1 tablespoon per day. Once your symptoms have abated, take 1 tablespoon of flax oil three times per week to support your intestinal function and promote healing of your intestines. This prescription's success is affected by how well you implement all the recommended dietary changes, too.

Kava Kava

Kava kava is derived from the roots of the kava kava plant (*Piper methysticum*). It relaxes the nervous system, reduces anxiety, and reduces or eliminates insomnia. Because it is so relaxing, it should not be taken before driving. Kava kava is available in tea bags, as a dried herb, and in pill form. To prepare a cup of tea, use 1 teaspoon of dried herb for every 1 cup of water. Place the herb and water in a saucepan, bring the water to a boil, then remove the saucepan from the flame and allow the herb to steep for 15–20 minutes. Strain out the herb and drink the tea as needed.

Milk Thistle

Milk thistle is derived from the common milk thistle plant (*Sylibum marianum*). It promotes healing of the liver and gall bladder, and helps reverse toxic liver damage from drugs. In fact, it is revered for its ability to regenerate the liver cells and promote healthy hepatic function. Milk thistle is widely available in natural foods stores in tea bags, as a dried herb, in pill form, and in tinctures. To prepare a cup of tea, use 1 teaspoon of dried herb for every 1 cup of water. Place the herb and water in a saucepan, bring the water to a boil, then remove the saucepan from the flame and allow the herb to steep for 15–20 minutes. Strain out the herb before serving. Drink 1 to 2 cups a day for a week, rest for a week, and then drink 1 or 2 cups a day again for up to a week.

Slippery Elm

Slippery elm is derived from the bark of the slippery elm tree *(Ulmus fulva)*. It soothes irritated mucous membranes and strengthens debilitated conditions. Slippery elm is available in tea bags, as a dried herb, and in pill form. To prepare a cup of tea, use 1 tablespoon of dried herb for every 1 cup of water. Place the herb and water in a saucepan, bring the water to a boil, then remove the saucepan from the flame and allow the herb to steep for 15–20 minutes. Strain out the herb and drink 1–2 cups per day.

Valerian

Valerian is derived from the root of the valerian plant *(Valeriana officinalis)*. It is very effective at calming anxiety and nervous tension. It relieves gas in the lower abdomen, calms spasms, and promotes deeper sleep. It is well known as a safe sleep aid. Valerian is widely available in natural foods stores in tea bags, as a dried herb, and as a tincture. To prepare a cup of tea, use 1 teaspoon of dried herb for every 1 cup of water. Place the herb and water in a saucepan, bring the water to a boil, then remove the saucepan from the flame and allow the herb to steep for 15 minutes. Strain out the herb and drink 1–3 cups per day.

Healing Lifestyle Practices

Daily life is really a string of behaviors, many of which we repeat, day in and day out. We get up at a certain hour and we perform certain activities every morning, every afternoon, and every evening. Our repeating behaviors form the familiar patterns of our lives, patterns we refer to as our "lifestyle." Imbedded in our lifestyle are the myriad practices we follow to cope with stress and negative emotions. Our lifestyle determines, for example, how well or how poorly we take care of our body; whether or not we regularly exercise, meditate, or pray; whether we spend time in nature; whether we write about our feelings on a regular basis; or whether we make a point of listening to uplifting music.

Our daily patterns have a tremendous impact on our health. Indeed, they either promote our health or diminish it. Because these patterns are so familiar to us, they tend to become invisible—that is, until our health falters or we begin to suffer from a serious illness.

Lifestyle plays an essential role in the healing of Crohn's, colitis, and other IBDs, in part because the health of our digestive tract is so easily affected by our emotions and particularly by stress. Therefore, we have to look at our lifestyle and make changes where appropriate. In this section, I will describe some of the lifestyle changes I hope you will make to promote your full recovery from IBD. Most of the behaviors discussed are activities I used to get well. Note that you do not have to adapt all of the behaviors I discuss. On the contrary, I encourage you to choose just what appeals to you and incorporate them into your daily life. This may mean that you will select only one or two of the behaviors. That's fine. Do what you can now and expand your health-promoting activities as your health and vitality improve. Allow me to make one general recommendation, however. I urge you to adopt two lifestyle practices that I believe will have immediate and dramatic impact on your life. The first is exercise, which I describe below. The second is some form of emotional or spiritual practice that can provide you with a direct experience of comfort and solace on a daily basis. When coupled with the macrobiotic dietary practices I have already described, these two activities—one yang, the other yin—can become the basis for a tremendous transformation in your health and overall way of living.

Exercise on a Regular Basis

There is no end to the physical benefits of exercise, it seems. Exercise improves the circulation throughout the body, boosts strength and muscle fitness, increases the amount of oxygen that is delivered to the cells, eliminates toxins, strengthens cardiovascular health, improves sleep, reduces stress, and elevates mood. As if all that were not enough, exercise is not something you need to do a lot of to reap rewards, as many people believe. A 20-minute daily walk at a moderate pace will get you all the benefits just mentioned. You can even just stroll around the block once, twice, or three times a day and see tremendous improvements. Every little bit you do has a significant impact on your life.

There is an endless variety of exercises you can enjoy that will improve your health—everything from yoga, bicycling, and swimming, to tennis, golf, and weight training—but the exercise with which I recommend you begin is walking. Walk at a pace that allows you to talk while walking without feeling out of breath. If you can talk easily, you are not placing too much stress on your heart, circulatory system, lungs, or muscles. As you walk, swing your arms gently from your shoulders and allow your hips to move freely. It's important not to push yourself too hard, especially if you have not exercised for some time and are out of shape. Start out walking for up to a mile and then gradually increase your distance to two miles, if you can.

Give Yourself a Body Rub

In addition to walking, I urge you to give yourself a body rub with a hand towel five or six days per week. Body rubs are especially good for people who are too weak to walk or do some other form of exercise.

To give yourself a body rub, make sure your body is dry. Dip a cotton towel in hot water and wring it out well. Fold the towel to make it two to four layers thick and scrub your dry body with it in a back and forth motion. Cover your entire body in an orderly manner, starting either at your head and face and working down to your feet, or vice versa. It should take you about 15 minutes to do it well. The object of the body rub is to make your skin red, which means you are promoting circulation throughout your body. Don't worry if your skin doesn't get red in the beginning; it will in time as the condition of your skin and circulatory system improves.

Body rubs deep-clean your skin, open your pores, and increase your circulation, blood flow, and the oxygenation of your cells. They also promote the cleansing of your lymph system and the flow of energy throughout your body. A good body rub will improve all the aspects of your physical, emotional, and mental health. Do your body rub first thing in the morning or right before going to bed.

Give Your Digestion Time and Energy to Heal

Refrain from eating or drinking at least three hours before retiring to bed for the night. This will give your body enough time to digest your dinner and take the stress off your stomach and intestines. While we sleep, our immune system utilizes the vitamins, minerals, and phytochemicals we ate during the day to address the wounds, infections, and conditions against which our body is struggling. It also accumulates toxins during the night to be expelled in the morning. In other words, our digestive system, kidneys, and liver regenerate during sleep. To facilitate this process, our whole body, including our digestive system, should be in a resting mode and not working during that time.

Chew, Chew, Chew

Of course, you should always sit while eating and assume a relaxed, centered attitude in preparation for your meal. Once you begin eating, chew every mouthful at least 50 times, on average, and between 150 and 200 times when your system needs deep healing. It is especially important to chew thoroughly during flare-ups.

You may find it difficult at first to chew a mouthful of food that much, since you will tend to swallow the food before you've chewed it even 50 times. You have to concentrate on what you are doing—namely eating and chewing—to keep the food in your mouth and chew it that many times. With practice, you'll discover that food tastes infinitely better when it is thoroughly chewed. By fully masticating food, you break it into very fine and tiny pieces, which takes the stress off your stomach and small intestine. You also make the nutrients in the food far more accessible to your small intestine, thus improving assimilation and enriching your blood, cells, and immune system with more nutrition.

The more you chew, of course, the more of your saliva will be mixed with the food. This will alkalize the food, which in itself will promote healing of the digestive tract. It will also cause far more digestive enzymes to be mixed with the food, thus further improving assimilation.

There are so many reasons to chew at least 50 times per mouthful, and at best 150 to 200 times per mouthful, but allow me to describe two more. When you chew your food thoroughly, you increase your relaxation while eating. As you relax, your body naturally releases its tension, which allows it to expand. That expansion makes your body better able to absorb the food and all of its nutrition and energy. As you chew and relax, your body focuses on receiving the food, which it does with far more gratitude and acceptance than if you just gobble your food down.

Finally, chewing makes you focus on the act of eating. This causes you to be more present as you eat. Try chewing a mouthful 150 times as an experiment and see what effect it has on your mood and consciousness. Thoroughly chewing my meal always causes me to feel much more balanced, centered, and in the moment. I feel more at peace and integrated within myself. I feel more alive within my own body. This gives me a unique sense of power, balance, and connectedness to my environment. Chewing becomes a kind of meditation, which makes eating a spiritual practice.

A special friend of mine made a "chewing bracelet" out of beads to help with the counting process. The bracelet contains 20 beads—18 small, one medium, and one large. To make the bracelet, take a piece of elastic string and string the large bead first. Next string nine of the small beads, follow with the medium bead, and finish with the remaining nine beads. Knot the ends of the string and place the bracelet on your wrist. When chewing, count 10 bites per bead until you make it all the way around for a total of 200 chews per bite. The medium bead indicates the halfway point in the chewing process. Counting your chewing this way definitely slows down eating and is well worth it for your intestines.

Practice Meditation

Meditation is the act of sitting peacefully and focusing your attention on an image, a prayer, a mantra, or a passage from literature or scripture, and allowing that object of your attention to relax your mind and body. Once your mind and body have achieved a state of deep relaxation, another aspect of your being—let's say your spirit or soul—is allowed to rise and infuse you with its own powers and influence. The relaxation of your body serves to quiet your mind, release your body from tension, and let the gentler aspects of your being emerge. At that point, your spirit can start to inform your being. It can fill your awareness with feelings and images of peace and beauty, which in turn can give you a deeper sense of faith and security. At that moment, you can enter into a state of deep healing.

The two primary keys to successful meditation, therefore, are to achieve a state of deep relaxation and to do this using an object that inspires you.

The image, mantra, inspirational passage, or object of your attention must be something that resonates with the inner you. Of course, the specific object will vary for all of us, depending upon our personal histories. I recommend that you work with an image that you create in your mind or an object such as a candle flame, a mantra, or a passage from scripture.

There are many images you can use that have been handed down through the centuries. You can picture being or conversing with a spiritual figure to whom you feel deeply connected, such as Jesus, Buddha, or Moses. You can do the same with a departed ancestor, such as a grandparent or parent, or even with a spiritual guide or angel. All these images can induce a state of deep relaxation and comfort.

A Health-Restoring Image Routine

The following is an ancient healing meditation that you can use to help boost your immune system and restore your health:

Sit in a peaceful place and imagine a diamond of light just above your head. Envision that diamond of light sending a beam of bright white light into the top of your head. Feel that light fill every one of your sense organs—your eyes, your nose, your ears, and your mouth—and infuse every cell in your head with light. Feel the light flow like a river down into your neck and shoulders, imbuing you with energy and life force. From your shoulders, feel it flow into your heart and fill your entire chest. Feel your heart open up and the light become stronger, more powerful, radiating up into your shoulders and down into your arms and fingers. Feel great beams of light flow from your fingertips. See the light pulsate with every beat of your heart. Feel it snake its way down into your small and large intestines, healing every inch of them. Feel it illuminate every cell with new life and vitality. Feel the main river of light flow into your reproductive organs, transforming them into pulsating, vital, life-imbued tissues. Feel every cell ablaze with light and life. Feel all your injuries, all your disorders, all your painful memories being released from your tissues as the light transforms your entire reproductive area. Now feel the light move down into your legs, slowly and powerfully, releasing all fatigue and restoring their energy, vitality, and lightness. Feel it flow into your feet and restore their vitality, lightness, and energy. Feel the light flow from the bottoms of your feet and toes down into the earth, anchoring you to the world. You are safe and secure, held by Mother Nature, and imbued with light, energy, and life. Every cell in your body is now healthier, more vital, more alive.

A Mantra

Mantras are words that have tremendous energy and power. They create a state of deep relaxation, peace, and faith. There are mantras from all traditions. If you choose to use a mantra, the most important thing is to find one that you can relate to and find inspiring and life-supporting. Among the most ancient mantras are:

- *Om,* an ancient Sanskrit word that means "universal sound."
- *Aum,* an extended version of *om.* It is pronounced by sounding out all three of the letters as syllables: A-U-M.
- *Su,* an ancient Japanese chant designed to open the heart.
- *Abba,* ancient Hebrew for "father."
- *Jesus, Mary, and Joseph,* the Holy family.
- *Nam myo ho renge kyo,* an ancient Buddhist chant designed to open and unify the seven chakras, or energy centers, of the body.
- *Amen,* Latin for "so be it," or "make it so."

A Passage from Scripture

There are many great sources of spiritual literature to provide any sort of representative sampling of powerful passages on which to meditate. For example, the Bible—both the Old and the New Testaments. My own orientation, as I have said in this book, is Christian, so allow me to share with you some of my own favorite passages from the Bible that I use for inspiration and strength while meditating.

- Corinthians 12:9: "My power is made perfect in weakness."
- Romans 8:28: "And we know that all things work together for good to those who love God, to those who are the called according to His purpose."
- Jeremiah 29:11: " For I know the plans I have for you, plans to prosper you and not to harm you, plans to give you hope and a future."
- 2 Corinthians 3:17: "The Lord is the spirit who gives life, and where He is there is freedom."
- Philippians 4:6, 4:7: "Be anxious for nothing, but in everything by prayer and supplication, with thanksgiving, let your requests be made known to God; and the peace of God, which surpasses all understanding, will guard your hearts and minds through Christ Jesus."
- Psalm 30:5: "Weeping may tarry for the night but joy comes with the morning."

- Philippians 4:13: "I can do all things through Christ who strengthens me." (This one is my favorite.)

I have found that just browsing through a great spiritual work is a source of tremendous inspiration and strength. Read individual passages and watch your life condition change.

Indulge in Music and Laughter

Surround yourself with uplifting music and songs that bring a smile to your face and lift your spirits. Socialize with people or participate in events that make you laugh. Studies show that people's endorphins, or "feel-good" chemicals, multiply when they are in a happy frame of mind. When a person is happy, healing is given a boost because the body is relieved from stress.

Get Sufficient Sleep

Don't underestimate the restorative power of deep sleep. Normal sleep consists of five stages. The brain progresses through each of these five stages every 90 minutes. Deep sleep occurs during the first part of the 90-minute sleep cycle, while rapid eye movement (REM) sleep, characterized by dreaming, occurs during the last part. The average person goes through four to six sleep cycles each night.

Our sleep needs change as we age. The length of the deep-sleep stage decreases as we mature. The amount of total sleep we need also decreases, dropping from 16 to 17 hours at birth to 10 to 12 hours at age four, to 9 to 10 hours at age ten. After adolescence, 8 hours per night becomes the average, gradually declining to about 6½ hours by old age. It is untrue that people need less sleep as they get older. Rather, we have less time to sleep at any one period, even nighttime, with napping during the day becoming more common and in turn compromising our ability to fall asleep at night.

While 8 hours is the average amount of sleep needed by adults, the actual amount varies among individuals. Many people in today's society deprive themselves of sleep due to their busy lives. If you are taking an IBD drug such as prednisone, your sleep patterns may be even more erratic. Continually getting less sleep can result in tiredness or even sleep deprivation. Sleep deprivation over time compromises the nervous system. The best way to determine the amount of sleep you need is to monitor how much sleep it takes for you to feel refreshed, effectively perform your daily activities, maintain your energy level throughout the day, and manage your stress levels effectively.

Try to get to sleep by 10:00 to 11:00 P.M. and to wake up by 7:00 A.M. The natural healing process takes place only during deep sleep and certain organs are regenerated only at certain hourly cycles during the night. Adjusting your sleep habits will help your body respond quicker to healing.

To help yourself fall asleep at night, promote a sleeping atmosphere before going to bed. One way to relax is to soak your feet in hot water for 3 to 10 minutes. Two to three times a week, take a hot bath. Adding a relaxing oil, such as lavender oil, to the water will further promote relaxation.

Have Body Work Done

"Body work" is a kind of umbrella term for the many forms of therapeutic massage currently practiced. Physical tension is the basis for many illnesses, in part because tension causes the muscles to go into spasm, which in turn prevents the optimal flow of blood, oxygen, nutrients, immune cells, and lymph to the tissues. Without these blood constituents, cells die, waste products accumulate, and organs begin to degenerate. A person with a healing touch—that is, someone whose touch causes the body to relax— is capable of taking those muscles out of spasm and promoting circulation to cells and tissues that have been deprived of those essential life ingredients.

Body work is especially important for people with Crohn's disease or other IBDs because we tend to experience excessive amounts of tension in our abdomen. This, of course, affects our digestive tract, especially the small and the large intestines.

More and more practitioners are practicing the various types of body work available today. Among the most widely available forms of body work are the following:

- *Acupressure.* A form of massage based on Chinese acupuncture in which acupuncture points are stimulated by finger manipulation to promote an increase in energy along a pathway, or meridian, to a specific organ. This is a highly effective form of massage and one that I highly recommend.
- *Alexander technique.* Created by F. Matthias Alexander, it focuses on the improvement of posture, which practitioners maintain controls to a great degree the respiratory, nervous, and muscular systems.
- *Feldenkrais method.* Also known as "awareness through movement," this is a form of physical therapy that involves gentle movements, healing touch, breathing techniques, and posture alignment to bring about physical and psychological transformation.
- *Jin shin jyutsu.* A system created by twentieth-century Japanese sage Jiro Murai that stimulates 26 points on the body known as "safety energy locks," which act as conductors of the life energy to specific organs, systems, and regions of the body.
- *Ohashiatsu.* A form of shiatsu created by Japanese teacher Waturo Ohashi.
- *Reflexology.* An ancient form of massage that stimulates various points on the feet that correspond with the organs and systems. The practice is based on principles similar to those of acupressure and shiatsu, in which the stimulated points send life energy—known in Chinese as *chi* and in Japanese as *ki*—to specific organs and thus promote healing.
- *Reiki.* A Tibetan form of the laying on of hands. Practitioners are trained to send life energy through their hands and into the body of their client, thus elevating the client's healing energy and promoting recovery.
- *Shiatsu.* The Japanese form of acupressure, or meridian massage, based on the same principles and techniques as acupressure.

- *Therapeutic touch.* A form of the laying on of hands developed by and scientifically studied by Dolores Kreiger, a nursing professor and practitioner. Kreiger demonstrated the effectiveness of therapeutic touch to boost the immune system and to increase the speed and thoroughness of healing.

These are but a handful of the many forms of healing massage that can make a profound difference in your life. Explore the kind of healing touch that appeals to you the most and see a practitioner regularly.

Visit a Psychological Counselor

Finally, I encourage people with Crohn's, colitis, or other forms of IBD to seek the help of a trained counselor and see him or her on a regular basis. There are so many emotions and life experiences that create tension in the abdomen and lower organs that lead to digestive disorders. Our organs hold onto inscriptions and patterns. These become stagnant over time and cause us stress. As our bodies begin to let go, our memories of old experiences, feelings, smells, sounds, will emerge to be released. I sought professional help from several counselors, all of whom provided me with some important insight and comfort. I urge you to do the same.

One of the most important things any human being can do is to seek the help of others. Whether it is a dietary counselor, a massage therapist, or a professional counselor, the simple act of opening ourselves up and asking for help begins the healing journey. Take up that path and you will be led to your answers.

14

Medical Options

Surgery is performed on people with Crohn's disease, ulcerative colitis, and other inflammatory bowel disorders when they do not respond to medical therapy or require an operation to correct a blockage, perforation, abscess, or bleeding. No matter how well performed, surgery is not a cure for IBD. Rather, it is a measure designed to mitigate the symptoms for a relatively short period of time. The reason: Crohn's and ulcerative colitis spread from diseased to healthy tissue. Even if the diseased tissue is removed, the underlying conditions that caused the disease remain in place, which means that healthy tissue will soon be infected. If medical intervention does not effect a remission, the disease will rage, as before, and require additional surgery. For many people, numerous operations are needed until vast tracts of the intestine are eliminated.

Many surgeries are performed because of fistulas or abscesses. A fistula is formed by a wave of inflammation passing through the intestines and into the surrounding fat. Sometimes the inflammed area has nowhere to drain. This causes an infection to develop and an abscess to form. Abscesses are characterized by pain, fever, and localized tenderness. They must be drained.

Crohn's disease does not raise the risk of cancer. However, tumor-causing cells in tissues from organs such as the spleen and lymph nodes have been found in patients who have had Crohn's disease for a long time. The malignancy can occur in both affected and non-affected areas of the small and large intestines. A tissue biopsy is the most common test done when any irregular cells are found.

Ulcerative colitis recurs after surgery in unresected segments of the colon. In most cases, the surgery involves a total colonectomy and is seen as a cure. The risk of cancer is much higher with ulcerative colitis. Individuals who have ulcerative colitis involving the entire colon or whose disease has lasted 10 or more years have an increased risk of developing cancer. This group of patients requires periodic surveillance, including frequent colonoscopy.

When it comes to surgery, it is important to carefully weigh the risks versus the benefits, since this is a lifelong decision. I have heard from young teenagers with Crohn's or colitis who were urged by their doctors to undergo a drastic surgical procedure after their first attack. The reason, said the doctors, was that the attacks would keep coming. Why not have the surgery now and get it over with at an early age?

In this chapter, I outline the surgical procedures and drugs used to treat IBDs medically. Through the years, the medications have improved, but nothing offered through standard medical treatment actually heals the underlying disease or can be considered a cure.

Surgical Options

The total removal of the colon can be viewed as a cure for ulcerative colitis. Once the colon isn't there, it cannot become infected or inflamed.

Surgery for ulcerative colitis can be an elective procedure or done in an emergency situation. The medical emergency situations include:

- *Perforation.* Also called peritonitis, perforation is when the ulceration in the colon extends through the wall, resulting in a hole. Air and stool can then leak into the abdomen, causing severe infection. If left untreated, perforation causes rapid deterioration and shock. It usually occurs only in severely ill patients. It is rare in Crohn's disease.

- *Bleeding.* Episodes of massive bleeding or hemorrhage are frightening to both patients and their families. Luckily, such episodes are experienced by only about 5 percent of patients. Once the source of the bleeding has been isolated, surgery can be performed on the affected segment of the bowel. Severe bleeding requiring emergency colonectomy is uncommon.

- *Fistulas and abscesses.* In many patients, the inflammation of Crohn's or ulcerative colitis will extend beyond the intestinal walls and into the surrounding fat, producing a fistula. The inflammation may make its way into another segment of the bowel, into another organ such as the bladder or abdomen, or into the colon wall near the rectum. Sometimes there will be no place for the inflamed cells to drain, causing an infection to build up until an abscess is formed. Abscesses must be drained. All fistulas are not equal in severity, so the condition is not an absolute indication for surgery.

- *Obstruction.* Obstruction usually shows up late in the course of Crohn's disease. After years of inflammation, the bowel will thicken and eventually narrow, so that food can no longer pass through.

- *Fulminant colitis.* Fulminant colitis is colitis that occurs very suddenly or is very severe. It is caused by severe diarrhea, bleeding, and fever. Some physicians wait for as few as five days for signs of improvement. Others may wait for up to 14 days before recommending a total colonectomy.

- *Toxic megacolon.* In megacolon, the colon loses its muscle tone, becoming dilated and elongated. This results in a high risk of perforation. Toxic megacolon is a complication of ulcerative colitis.

The elective surgical situations include:

- *Intractability.* Intractability is the difficulty of managing your disease. It is different for each patient. Some people who are unresponsive to medical treatment and experiencing toxicity from their medications that is significantly affecting their lives may choose surgery because they see it as an end to their suffering.
- *Risk of Cancer.* Individuals who have ulcerative colitis involving the entire colon and have had the disease for 10 years or longer have an increased risk of developing colon cancer. If they are found to have severe dysplasia (cell changes that may lead to cancer), they may opt to have surgery, since dysplasia indicates that cancer is either present or will develop in the near future.
- *Crohn's disease.* Surgery never cures Crohn's disease. Crohn's frequently recurs after surgery. The indications for surgery vary depending on the site of the disease, its complications, and its responsiveness to medication. However, emergency surgery may be required in some cases even before a diagnosis is made. These patients have the classic signs of appendicitis: fever and pain in the right lower abdomen even if the appendix is normal.

Surgical Procedures

There are four surgical procedures generally performed on persons with IBD. These are:

- *Total colonectomy.* A total colonectomy is the removal of the entire colon. Over one million Americans have had this procedure. A small opening called a stoma is created in the abdominal wall to allow waste to be eliminated from the body. A pouch is attached at this stoma and worn at the side to collect the waste. The stoma is located in the right lower quadrant of the abdomen, since this is where the ileum is located. The pouch is emptied by the patient as necessary. A total colonectomy usually requires a hospital stay of eight to

12 days. Recovery takes roughly two weeks and is determined by how well the patient is passing waste into the pouch. Follow-up support is needed to educate the patient in the care of the stoma and pouch.

- *Partial colonectomy.* A partial colonectomy is the removal of only the diseased section of the colon. The rectum is left intact and is resected, or attached, to the healthy part of the colon.

- *J-pouch.* Individuals with ulcerative colitis are candidates for this operation, but those with Crohn's are not. This is because Crohn's usually involves the small intestines and this procedure involves stretching the small intestine to the anal canal to create a new rectum. The J-pouch operation is performed in two stages. In the first stage, the diseased colon and the rectal lining are removed and the ileum is joined to the anal canal using a pouch created from adjacent loops of the ileum. In the second stage, performed about two months after the first, the ileostomy is closed. A small incision is made around the ileostomy. The stoma in the bowel is sewn closed and the ileum is returned to the inside of the abdomen. The patient is fed intravenously for three to four days, or until the bowels start to move again. The hospital stay is usually about seven days after the second surgery. Regular activities can be resumed roughly six weeks after the operation. About 25 to 30 percent of patients experience slight fecal spotting or staining, which takes about five years to begin decreasing. In the weeks or months after the operation, some patients develop an inflammation in the pouch. This may be due to an overgrowth of bacteria in the pouch.

- *Kock pouch.* The kock pouch procedure is an alternative to the standard colonectomy. The advantage is that an external appliance is not required to collect the waste matter. Instead, an internal reservoir is created out of several loops of intestines. This internal pouch is cleaned periodically by inserting a catheter through an abdominal stoma, which can be covered by a single bandage. The kock pouch procedure is best done for ulcerative colitis but is not justified for Crohn's. Crohn's tends to spread in the small intestines and could therefore affect the surgically created pouch. About 15 percent of patients require some form of revisional surgery, usually for incontinence, prolapse, or skin strictures.

Medication Options

The first goal of treatment for IBD is to control inflammation, which in turn will bring relief of abdominal pain, diarrhea, and rectal bleeding. All the prescription drugs used to treat IBD have frequent and serious side effects, and thus require ongoing medical monitoring. Moreover, the medications are generally used for extended periods of time. This, of course, increases the chances of suffering adverse reactions.

Drug treatments for IBD do not address the underlying causes of the disease, but instead attempt to reduce the severity of the symptoms. Their true intention, in fact, is to mask the symptoms of the disease. In time, the symptoms become more severe, requiring stronger doses of the medication, until surgery becomes necessary.

There are numerous over-the-counter medications used to treat IBD symptoms. They are designed to treat the diarrhea, cramping, gas, bloating, and other discomforts due to indigestion. These drugs are symptomatic medicines that help with mild to moderate symptoms of Crohn's and colitis, mainly diarrhea. They can be taken orally before meals or at bedtime as the label directions indicate. These over-the-counter medications include Pepto Bismol, Lomotil, Imodium, and Paregoric.

There are also a number of drugs available by prescription for mild to moderate symptoms of IBD. These drugs include codeine, deodorized tincture of opium (DTO), dicyclomine (Bentyl), hyoscyamine (Levsin), questran (Cholestyramine), and Claritin, an antihistamine that is effective when ulcerative colitis symptoms are triggered by allergies, mainly to pollen. The potential side effects of these medications are drowsiness.

There are also a number of stronger prescription drugs used to treat Crohn's disease, ulcerative colitis, and other IBDs.

Mesalamine

Mesalamine, also known as 5-ASA, affects the colon and is most often used to treat constipation and abdominal gas. It has an anti-inflammatory effect on the mucosal lining of the large intestine. For some people with ulcerative colitis or Crohn's, 5-ASA can reduce the symptoms of the disease and help to maintain remission. It may also help prevent recurrence of the symptoms after surgery.

Mesalamine is available under three brand names: Asacol and Pentasa, which are taken orally, and Rowasa, which is taken by enema or suppository. All may cause allergies or a worsening of both colitis and Crohn's symptoms. They have also been found to cause kidney damage and hair loss. When used for an extended period of time, Rowasa may cause rectal irritation.

Sulfasalazine

Sulfasalazine is taken orally. It is used for mild to moderate Crohn's and ulcerative colitis. It is designed to reduce the symptoms and, for some, helps to maintain remission. Its potential side effects include rash, anemia, low sperm count, headache, nausea, vomiting, and GI distress. Its severe side effects include lung, liver, and bone marrow toxicity. Most of these side effects seem to be related. Because of the way sulfasalazine is metabolized by the body, it prevents the proper absorption of folic acid in the small intestine. The most common brand of sulfasalazine is Azulfidine.

Olsalazine

Taken orally, olsalazine is used to treat mild to moderate ulcerative colitis. It is designed to reduce the symptoms and attempt to effect a remission. It seems to be as effective as sulfasalazine in treating IBD symptoms. It is often first taken in small doses, which are then gradually adjusted. Its potential side effects are diarrhea and allergy. Olsalazine is available under the trade names of Dipentum, Asacol, and Pentasa. Asacol is coated with acrylic resins to protect the drug from being dissolved by stomach acids. It is released further down the digestive tract into the terminal ileum and colon. Pentasa is also coated and released in a time-dependent manner into the small intestine or colon.

Corticosteroids

Among the most commonly prescribed medications for Crohn's and colitis, the corticosteroids are steroids, or hormones that resemble cortisol, which is secreted by the adrenal gland when the body is under stress. The corticosteroids—including prednisone, methylprednisolone, and hydrocortisone—are designed to reduce inflammation, control symptoms, and induce remission. They are not effective at preventing the onset of IBD symptoms. They have many moderate to severe side effects, including osteoporosis, hypertension (high blood pressure), diabetes, cataracts, lowered potassium levels, rapid aging of the skin, acne, hip necrosis, and psychological problems. They are also appetite stimulants by the direct action of the steroid on the brain. The corticosteroids improve the mood and encourage a sense of well-being because they affect the emotional centers of the brain. They therefore mask severe disease. Because of this, their use must be monitored carefully. These drugs are taken orally, intravenously, and rectally, either as suppositories, enemas, or foams.

Immunomodulators and Immunosuppressives

Among the many things the immune system does is create inflammation as a way of defeating disease. Immunomodulators and immunosuppressives control or suppress the immune system, thus stopping the body's defenses from creating inflammation and attacking diseased tissues in the small and the large intestines. The drugs work by reducing the number of white blood cells and immune factors. This lowers the body's ability to create inflammation and allows the doctor to lower the dosage of the steroid.

Immunomodulators and immunosuppressives are used to treat both Crohn's and ulcerative colitis, especially when fistulas occur. The potential side effects are pancreatitis, allergies, allergic pneumonia, fever, weakened immunity, a lowered white count, increased vulnerability to infections, and liver toxicity. Among the immunomodulators and immunosuppressives are azathioprine (Immuran), which is taken orally; 6-mercaptopurine (6-MP or Purinethol), which is taken orally; cyclosporine (Neoral), which is taken orally or administered by IV; and methotrexate (Rheumatrex), which is taken orally or administered by injection.

Sandimmune, which is administered orally or intravenously, is used for severe ulcerative colitis, severe Crohn's, and fistulas. The potential side effects of long-term use include kidney toxicity, liver toxicity, unwanted hair growth, tremors, high blood pressure, and tumors.

Thalidomide (Thalomid), which is taken orally, is used for Crohn's disease that is moderate to severe. It is also used for fistulas and may prevent Crohn's flare-ups. It is used for its sedative and anti-inflammatory properties. However, many people feel that its severe side effects far outweigh these benefits. The side effects include severe congenital abnormalities in offspring, drowsiness, and nerve damage to the legs and arms. The side effects of long-term use are unknown.

TNF-Alpha Inhibitors

TNF-alpha inhibitors are used to treat moderate Crohn's disease and fistulas, and to prevent flare-ups. The most common TNF-alpha inhibitor used for Crohn's, colitis, and other IBDs is infliximab (Remicade). Infliximab blocks the action of protein known to activate inflammation. It is given intravenously or as an intramuscular injection. The IV infusion takes two hours and is followed by an hour-long observation period. Benedryl and

Tylenol are usually administered before the infusion is started to prevent fever and allergic reaction. Patients with Crohn's who do not have fistulas receive a single infusion, while those with fistulas receive three infusions spread over a number of weeks. Infliximab reduces symptoms within four weeks. An abscess may develop around the fistula about eight to 16 weeks after the final infusion.

The potential side effects of infliximab are an allergic reaction to the infusion, serum sickness, joint inflammation, and pain. The severe side effects include lymphoma and rheumatoid arthritis. Some people develop what is referred to as double-stranded DNA, which is found in the autoimmune disease lupus.

Antibiotics

Antibiotics are used to treat infections, fistulas, abscesses, perforations, secondary infections, and flare-ups. They are administered intravenously when the disease is severe and when there is a complication such as toxic megacolon. Their potential side effects include drowsiness, diarrhea, allergic reactions, vomiting, headache, nerve damage to the legs and arms, weakness, vaginitis, and thrush. Among the antibiotics used for IBDs are ciprofloxacin (Cipro), which is taken orally and intravenously, and metronidazole (Flagyl), which is taken orally.

Medications can have an important and highly therapeutic function in the treatment of Crohn's, colitis, and other IBDs. Taken for short periods, they can help people emerge from crises and can restore the body to a more balanced condition, at which point longer-term and deeper solutions, such as diet and lifestyle changes, can be used effectively. I have long wanted to see a combination of medical therapy and macrobiotics used to treat IBDs. For that to happen, however, we will need farsighted physicians who know how to administer standard medical treatments, while teaching people how to use food to create long-term healing.

Conclusion

In this book, I have tried to show you how I overcame a very serious inflammatory bowel disorder, namely Crohn's disease, and how you can do it, too. Many so-called experts told me along the way that Crohn's is incurable and **that what I was eating had nothing to do with it.** The only way I could ever manage the illness successfully was with powerful drugs and surgery. Those who told me that had very authoritative credentials. They were highly educated. Yet, they were wrong.

Looking back, I realize now that all I had was a belief in myself, a belief in those who tried to help me, and the willingness to trust my own experience. The macrobiotic diet and lifestyle had a profound impact on my life. It affected my symptoms and eventually helped me overcome my disorder. Along the way, I allowed my experience and my faith to guide me. My experience of the diet and lifestyle was what I needed most to sustain my trust in this program. I saw how much good it was doing me. No one could take that away from me.

The most difficult part about this practice is how simple it is. It is basic common sense. Therefore, it takes intentional thinking, dedication, and implementation. It is not magic. In a society that expects everything fixed quickly without much personal input, being the steward of your own health becomes a major challenge. Society today has a "magic pill" mentality. If it's not a pill, shot, or drink, we don't want to spend too much time thinking about it. We have luxurized saving time, but at what cost, if we are too sick to enjoy life? There are a number of influences that helped weaken our immune system and break down our health. Therefore, there is no one magic anything that will make us healthy. If we deny the cause, we also deny the cure.

Good health is created through a natural lifestyle. Our bodies function in a healthy state when we align with nature. Doing this includes more than just eating the right foods. Food is definitely the first step, since it's our nourishment. And I mean real food— God-made food, not manmade food. The closer the food is to its natural state, its raw unrefined form, the higher its quality and the stronger its life force. When a person resorts to ingesting stimulants of any kind or highly refined foods, he or she aborts the regeneration of the body.

It finally became clear to me that if I take care of myself, my body, my mind, and my spirit, I will have health, energy, time, and love to be of service to others and to be fruitful.

The macrobiotic lifestyle takes time, commitment, dedication, and a gut desire to want to not just be well, but to experience true healing. Yes, I said "time." When you weigh out how much time you spend in bed feeling bad, dragging yourself through the day feeling like you've accomplished only half of what you wanted to accomplish, and going to doctor appointment after doctor appointment, you'll realize that a few hours in the kitchen is well worth it. As I started putting the time into my new natural lifestyle, the energy I gained was incredible. And yes, I began having more time available to me. The time to start is now, because the power is in the present moment. Macrobiotics taught me that the body wants to be in a healthy state. Healing is the rule, not the exception. The body's tendency is to regenerate and maintain balance in order to experience health. When the body is provided with the proper tools, healing happens from within. Macrobiotics is the compass, the tool of navigation that leads to the whole, big, large, "macro" life.

As I have tried to show, I had many setbacks and made many

mistakes along the way. But I always had an intuitive awareness that I was on the right track and that somehow I was being led, or directed, by a Greater Good, **that my prayers were being answered.** I *behaved* my way to success. By applying myself to my daily activity, the results were evident.

I offer you this book in the same spirit. Use this diet and lifestyle with all your intelligence, willpower, and capacity to reflect on your own experience. Be aware of what is working for you and what isn't in all areas of your life: the **physical, emotional, and spiritual realm.** Get help whenever you need it, both from a medical doctor and from a macrobiotic counselor you trust. But most of all, apply yourself fully to your own healing. Let your spirit and the influences of a Higher Power guide you to your goal of health and rebirth and that quality of healing you can never get from a pill.

> If we leave Nature alone, she recovers gently from the disorder into which she has fallen.
> It is our anxiety, our impatience, which spoils all; and nearly all men die of their remedies, not of their diseases.
>
> —Moliere

> Accept everything with great pleasure and thanks. Accept misfortune like happiness, disease like health, poverty like prosperity. And if you do not like it and cannot stand it, refer to your Universal Compass, The Unique Principle. There you will find the best direction. Everything that happens to you is what you lack. All that is antagonistic or unbearable is complimentary. The person who embraces his or her antagonist is the happiest person.
>
> —George Ohsawa

Bibliography

Aihara, Herman. *Acid and Alkaline.* Oroville, CA: George Ohsawa Macrobiotic Foundation, 1986.

Anderson, Richard, N.D., N.M.D. *Cleanse & Purify Thyself Book 1.5.* Mt. Shasta, CA: Triumph, 1998.

Ber, Leonid, M.D.; and Gazella, Karolyn A. *Activate Your Immune System.* Green Bay, WI: IMPAKT Communications, Inc, 1998.

Brandt, Lawrence J.; and Steiner-Grossman, Penny. *Treating IBD: A Patient's Guide to the Medical and Surgical Management of Inflammatory Bowel Disease.* New York, NY: Raven Press, 1989.

Carter-Scott, Cherie, Ph.D. *If Life Is a Game, These Are the Rules.* New York, NY: Bantam Doubleday Dell Publishing, 1998.

Degenhardt, Katherine. *Praying God's Promises.* Nashville, TN: SEED Publishers, 1999.

Dufty, William. *Sugar Blues.* New York, NY: Warner Communications Company, 1975.

Esko, Wendy; and Kushi, Aveline. *Introducing Macrobiotic Cooking.* Tokyo, Japan: Japan Publications, 1978.

Goldberg, Burton. *Alternative Medicine: The Definitive Guide.* Tiburon, CA: Future Medicine Publishing, Inc, 1993.

Haas, Elson M., M.D. *Staying Healthy with the Seasons.* Berkeley, CA: Celestial Arts, 1981.

Henner, Marilu. *Total Health Makeover.* New York, NY: HarperCollins Publishers, 1998.

Kushi, Aveline; and Jack, Alex. *Complete Guide to Macrobiotic Cooking.* New York, NY: Warner Communications Company, 1985.

Kushi, Michio. *Macrobiotic Home Remedies.* Tokyo, Japan and New York, NY: Japan Publications, 1985.

Kushi, Michio. *Natural Healing Through Macrobiotics.* Tokyo, Japan: Japan Publications, 1978.

Lopez, D.A., M.D.; Williams, R.M., M.D., Ph.D.; and Miehlke, K., M.D. *Enzymes: The Fountain of Life.* Munchen, Germany: The Neville Press, 1994.

Malkmus, George H. *Why Christians Get Sick.* Shippensburg, PA: Treasure House, 1995.

McKenna, Marlene; and Monte, Tom. *When Hope Never Dies.* New York, NY: Kensington Books, 2000.

Muramoto, Naboru. *Healing Ourselves.* New York, NY: Avon, 1973.

Nussbaum, Elaine. *Recovery: From Cancer to Health Through Macrobiotics.* Tokyo, Japan, and New York, NY: Japan Publications, 1986.

Ody, Penelope. *The Complete Medicinal Herbal.* New York, NY: Dorling Kindersley Limited, 1993.

Oski, Frank A., M.D. *Don't Drink Your Milk!* Brushton, NY: TEACH Services, 1996.

Parham, Barbara. *What's Wrong with Eating Meat?* Denver, CO: Ananda Marga Publications, 1979.

Pirello, Christina. *Cook Your Way to the Life You Want.* New York, NY: Berkley Publishing, 1999.

Shuman, Sandy. *Macrobiotic Desserts.* Los Angeles, CA: Dictionart, 1981.

Stanchich, Lino. *Macrobiotic Healing Secrets: Volume 1.* Asheville, NC: Healthy Products, 2000.

Stanchich, Lino. *Power Eating Program: You Are How You Eat.* Coconut Grove, FL: Healthy Products Publisher, 1989.

Ticciati, Laura; and Ticciati, Robin, Ph.D., *Genetically Engineered Foods. Are They Safe? You Decide.* Los Angeles, CA: Keats Publishing, 1998.

Turner, Kristina. *The Self-Healing Cookbook.* Vashon Island, WA: Earthtones Press, 1987.

Wood, Rebecca. *The New Whole Foods Encyclopedia.* New York, NY: Penguin Books, 1999.

Index